THE NEW
WORLD *of*
SELF-HEALING

About the Author

Bente Hansen is a healer, spiritual counselor, Reiki master, channeler, and ordained minister. She was a columnist for Australia's *Conscious Living* magazine and contributes to the *Sedona Journal of Emergence*. She has a background in education and has conducted numerous workshops and seminars. Visit her website at www.dynamicenergyhealing.net.

To Write to the Author

If you wish to contact the author or would like more information about this book, please write to the author in care of Llewellyn Worldwide and we will forward your request. Both the author and publisher appreciate hearing from you and learning of your enjoyment of this book and how it has helped you. Llewellyn Worldwide cannot guarantee that every letter written to the author can be answered, but all will be forwarded. Please write to:

Bente Hansen
℅ Llewellyn Worldwide
2143 Wooddale Drive, Dept. 0-7387-0889-5
Woodbury, MN 55125-2989, U.S.A.

Please enclose a self-addressed stamped envelope for reply,
or $1.00 to cover costs.
If outside U.S.A., enclose international postal reply coupon.

Many of Llewellyn's authors have websites with additional information and resources. For more information, please visit our website at www.llewellyn.com.

THE NEW

Bente

Hansen

WORLD *of*

SELF-HEALING

Awakening

the Chakras

&

Rejuvenating

Your Energy Field

Llewellyn Publications
Woodbury, Minnesota

First Edition
Second Printing, 2007

Book design by Steffani Chambers
Cover design by Ellen Dahl
Cover photo © 2006 by BrandXPictures
Llewellyn is a registered trademark of Llewellyn Worldwide, Ltd.
Interior illustrations by Llewellyn Art Department.

Library of Congress Cataloging-in-Publication Data
Hansen, Bente.
    The new world of self-healing : awakening the chakras & rejuvenating your energy
field / Bente Hansen. -- 1st ed.
      p. cm.
    Includes bibliographical references (p.   ).
    ISBN-13: 978-0-7387-0889-8
    ISBN-10: 0-7387-0889-5
      1. Chakras. 2. Healing. 3. Self-care, Health. I. Title.

    RZ999.H3622 2006
    615.8'51--dc22

Llewellyn Worldwide does not participate in, endorse, or have any authority or responsibility concerning private business transactions between our authors and the public.

    All mail addressed to the author is forwarded but the publisher cannot, unless specifi-
cally instructed by the author, give out an address or phone number.

    Any Internet references contained in this work are current at publication time, but the
publisher cannot guarantee that a specific location will continue to be maintained. Please
refer to the publisher's website for links to authors' websites and other sources.

Note: The author and publisher of this book are not responsible in any manner whatso-
ever for any injury that may occur through following the instructions contained herein.
It is recommended that before beginning the techniques, you consult with your physi-
cian to determine whether you are medically, physically, and mentally fit to undertake
this course of practice.

Llewellyn Publications
A Division of Llewellyn Worldwide, Ltd.
2143 Wooddale Drive, Dept. 0-7387-0889-5
Woodbury, MN 55125-2989, U.S.A.
www.llewellyn.com

Printed in the United States of America

Also by Bente Hansen

Messages from Beyond (2001)

CONTENTS

Preface

"If you don't know the way,
walk slowly."

Signs and messages usually arrive unexpectedly, without fanfare or expectation. This was the case with my preparations for a one-day workshop. I was exploring topics of importance for inclusion and was astounded by the realization that there was substantial information, enough for a book. That awareness was the conception of this book. Since that time, there have been moments of both elation and exhaustion as the process of this book's gestation has unfolded.

My interest in health and wellness spans over thirty years. Extensive reading and adhering to an array of diet and fitness regimes reflect a belief that good health is possible and can be a reality for anyone until it is time to depart the physical body. However, major life changes in the early '90s provided an opportunity for me to explore healing on a deeper level. I was guided to leave behind a traditional career and delve into a field that was totally foreign on the conscious level, yet seemingly comfortable and natural in another way.

As a healing arts practitioner, I see clients experiencing a vast range of conditions. Over time it became obvious that there were limited benefits in the healing support given to individuals. Real and lasting wellness seemed elusive, as no sooner was one condition healed than another would invariably manifest. This resulted in considerable reflection and questioning on my part, as I sought to make sense out of what was observed time and again. Yet on another level I knew that it is possible to maintain vitality and fitness right up until the time of departure —and that conviction remains steadfast.

As a consequence of ongoing questioning and searching, it has become apparent that good health and wellness depend on more than adhering to a healthy diet, exercising regularly, and having a positive attitude. There are many factors that contribute to vitality and quality of life. Each factor is a critical aspect of the whole healing process. The factors discussed and explored in this book are all vitally important for attaining and maintaining wellness. Some will be familiar and others may not. Obviously, as this book covers an extensive range of issues, it is not possible to include an in-depth analysis of each factor contributing to wellness. These are all amply researched and discussed elsewhere by other authors.

It is my intention to create awareness of a multifaceted approach for achieving healing on a deeper level. Therefore I have drawn together the understanding gained from years of interest in the field and from work undertaken with clients. A large portion of this understanding has occurred through my personal inner journey, where the nature of truth, reality, and the meaning of life have been extensively explored. As you will discover, my guidance from other dimensions has been my teacher for some years now. It is their wisdom that guides my sharing of the perspective on healing contained in this book.

Through regular meditation practice and an intensely focused determination to achieve greater understanding, a path of spiritual seeking seemed a viable option to explore. It was also the path of least resistance, as every other potential avenue for creating meaning in my life was fraught with obstacles! Adhering to a path of seeking spiritual awareness and growth was not without difficulty either. However, it became apparent from the very beginning that this was a learning process. The obvious rewards were quickly evident through increasing feelings of wellness and peace.

During many years spent working in the education sector, the advantages of applying the spiral curriculum to learning became apparent. This approach involves teaching a basic concept and then enabling the student to gain proficiency through practice. When the student is ready, that basic concept is expanded to encompass additional information. This in turn is further absorbed and internalized by the student. Learning increases in gradients as mastery is achieved, with new knowledge being incorporated and integrated with previous learning. My spiritual learning progresses similarly.

For some people seeking greater knowledge of spiritual wisdom, the obvious place to learn is from books and teachers. A great deal of my learning was acquired in my healing room, in meditations, during sleep when lucid dreaming would occur, and through interactions and communication with spirit beings from other dimensions. It took time and practice to become accustomed to this way of learning. Initially I sought verification or proof of whatever was shared, though in time my trust increased due to unsought corroboration and other synchronous events.

An explanation of the energy model shown by my teachers from other dimensions is detailed in section 1. This energy model was totally unfamiliar when it was first revealed. Over a period of time, the pieces came together and I was able to view this model from a holistic and integrated perspective. My teachers cleverly employed the spiral curriculum approach in their teaching, thereby reducing the possibility of incredulity or disbelief on my part.

When doing energy work on clients, I usually close my eyes, relax, and feel the movement of energy. Closing the eyes is a means used to eliminate distractions and to concentrate fully on whatever is happening within the client and the energy flow that is occurring. During this time my mind is completely clear of chatter, a state that has been achieved due to regular meditation practice. This enables me to feel the movement of energy and its differing frequencies. There are instances where images come to mind. These images often relate to energy and its flow. Gradually I came to see images that were linear and represented the energy grid that is described in chapter 4. Initially the meaning was unclear. However, as these images continued to appear, additional information was revealed. This was delivered via regular channeling and from the increasing detail shown in the images.

There were unexpected instances when visual images would demonstrate that this energy structure exists in absolutely everything. One day, when walking with a friend, we stopped at a park and he went to use the restroom. As I sat on a bench, I quietly relaxed my mind and observed the paving. Almost immediately my fingertips began tingling, an indication that energy work was in progress. By then it had become commonplace to undertake energy healing on the earth. In this relaxed state, I saw lines that were distorted, and within a few seconds they straightened and connected beautifully into the structure described clearly in this book.

What is the purpose of this energy model that has been shown? In time I came to understand its role in the healing process. This is energy at a subatomic level, for want of a better description. Illness occurs subtly and gradually. Its initial effect is on the subatomic composition of the body. Similarly, healing can only take place when there is healing of the subatomic energy system. The more I saw and worked with the energy system, the clearer the connection between it and the healing process became. It is this connection that is detailed in this book.

Section 1 explores the energy model and contains an explanation of its operation and functioning. It includes a perspective on health and healing that extends beyond the Western medicine model currently adopted and advocated. Section 2 contains practical information regarding basic changes that can be made to daily life for creating good health in terms of diet, exercise, and meditation. Included are chapters on the power of thought, reality creation, and releasing fears. Section 3 focuses on the inner, or spiritual, aspect essential for healing on a deeper level.

This book has been written because of a realization that occurred while I was undertaking preparations for a one-day workshop. It was obviously time to share in writing what had previously been shared with clients, friends, and participants in workshops. In addition, the morning following the workshop I awoke and the first words uttered were, "I have to write a book." Those words were spoken aloud with no conscious intent on my part and were another clear message.

A Learning Tool

The human body is incredibly complex, and each person exhibits a unique biochemistry, depending on lifestyle experiences and genetic blueprint. Therefore, each reader will respond to the information, strategies, and visualizations shared in this book and the accompanying CD according to the perceptions, beliefs, and health status he or she holds. Realistically, there is no one clear-cut and simple health strategy that can be prescribed and applied successfully for every individual or every situation. Health and wellness are as much a state of mind as they are a physical state of being.

This book is not intended for use as a medical compendium. If you have a medical condition that is being treated, it is important to follow the advice given by your health practitioner. However, you may find several strategies or explanations that may be helpful in dealing with your condition on another level. And, with application, this may actually ameliorate symptoms and increase well-being over time.

The theme of self-healing underpins the three distinctly different sections of the book. The background information contained in section one is essential to the understanding and application of the suggested strategies and visualizations that are outlined throughout the book. Realistically, the ways in which you utilize the information will be dependent upon your particular situation and needs.

The book has been written with two purposes in mind. First, I am sharing my experiences, perspective, and insights on how the healing process operates at a subtle level and also how specific life (energy) factors result in the creation of illness. While there may be some similarity in what is presented with information that is offered by other authors, I feel the energy model described here is vastly different from anything depicted elsewhere. I recommend that you take time to familiarize yourself with this model and its application and apply it to every aspect of your life.

Second, the book is a useful resource designed to be used as a tool for creating effective and lasting changes to health and well-being. It may be beneficial to initially read the book thoroughly. Allow yourself time to digest concepts and exercises that resonate with your life issues. Then, when you are ready to begin implementing some of the strategies and visualizations, select those that are relevant.

If, for example, you've become aware of the need to make changes to your thinking and attitude, it may be worthwhile to work through chapters 15 to18 in a consecutive manner. Or, if your life feels as though it is out of balance and stress is a constant factor, the chapters in section two are well worth exploring in depth. Often, making simple but effective changes in practical ways can result in increased feelings of inner calm and balance and a reduction in daily stresses.

Take time to implement the appropriate exercises in order to ensure that desired improvements are well rehearsed and integrated into your daily lifestyle. It may even be beneficial to supplement the exercises, whether from the book or the accompanying CD, with further in-depth reading on a particular subject in order to fully understand the relevance of particular concepts. For example, if you choose to learn meditation to reduce stress reactions, it would most likely be useful to read comprehensive books on the subject in addition to joining a class.

Once you are familiar with exercises relevant to your situation and have put them into practice, you may find that pleasing results are achieved with some of the strategies while others do not offer the same obvious results. Be patient with yourself and the routine you establish to create the desired changes. Often improvement is gradual and subtle, and only upon reflection does it becomes apparent that great progress has actually been made.

It is also important to feel comfortable in undertaking any of the exercises. Allow intuition to be your inner guide. You will instinctively feel comfortable doing some of the exercises and not others. At a later time when you have assimilated earlier learning, it may be appropriate to explore strategies that initially appeared daunting and uncomfortable. It is then likely you will derive benefit from undertaking those exercises that earlier appeared too challenging. Work at your own pace at all times and be selective about the exercises you choose. Where you instinctively feel it is appropriate to your needs to change the wording or to either add or delete some of the steps, allow your inner knowing to guide you in how best to apply the strategies and visualizations.

I recommend that you allow time for the integration of new learning. Set realistic goals so that you do not end up feeling pressured and impatient with your efforts. For example, when it is second nature to have full mindfulness of your every word and thought, it is likely that full integration of the concepts and exercises in chapters 15 through 18 has taken place. In the meantime, remind yourself whenever you experience a slippage that you are a work in progress. It may take months of diligent application to create the changes in well-being you seek.

Accept that the information in this book is intended as a guide to assist you to create the wellness, abundance, and joyfulness that is your birthright. It is not intended as a "do" and "don't do" compendium. Its usefulness as a reference tool may last several months or years, depending upon your interest and needs.

As you read the information shared in this book, allow your mind to explore the concepts, suggestions, and exercises. Reflect on them. Where possible, take time to put into practice some of the visualization exercises and strategies that may be especially relevant. I encourage you to use this book as a resource to be referred to as situations and issues arise in your life. You will take from it whatever is needed at any particular time.

Section	**ENERGY**
One	**MODEL**

CHAPTER ONE

The Beauty
of a Rose

*"We must be willing to get rid of the life we've planned,
so as to have the life that is waiting for us."*
—Joseph Campbell—

The beauty of a rose never diminishes, even long after the bloom has faded and all that is left is the husk of what once was. The beauty of it remains, for in time, after it has withered upon the bush, there comes to replace it yet another bloom, one of equally stunning beauty. Even after the magnificence of each bloom begins to fade, there is still a lingering scent. The beauty remains though the flower itself may not. That is the nature of you, of your soul. The beauty is always there regardless of what may happen in life. The beauty is undimmed and untarnished. In many instances, other aspects temporarily cover the beauty.

The journey of life itself creates difficulties within the human body. The daily hardships and challenges that confront the individual begin to take their toll, and so this kernel of beauty, this grain of truth at times becomes submerged beneath the many layers of grime, confusion, and pain that rest upon it. There comes a time when an individual may indeed believe they are no more than a grubby speck of dirt. As they look into their body, they may see physical ailments. Especially as the years encroach, there tends to be an increasing number of conditions and illnesses that beset the human physiology.

It is indeed not an easy task to see the inherent beauty beneath a body that is often crippled or gnarled with physical pain. It is interesting to observe, however, that underlying this, the spirit is indomitable. Human nature, being what it is, tends to rise to the surface with an acceptance of the status quo—not only acceptance but with it adjustments and justification for what is occurring physically. It is as if the spirit knows that in spite of the physical limitations and hardships it experiences, there is always underneath, at the very core center, something that is deeper, stronger, and enduring.

The other layers that build up over time are those of emotional and mental pain. The anguish these create ultimately within the physical body is considerable. With both emotional and mental pain there come strong beliefs and perceptions about how life really is. Life does not start off being this difficult but through the many experiences, interactions, and the deeply held beliefs that are taken on during embodiment, the human body becomes a vessel of pain. It carries this pain around it, very much like a shell, so that whatever else occurs in life, it can only further add to what already is there.

It would be inspiring to observe humanity shedding this pain. It would be a delight to see and feel the releasing of this pain. It is not necessary to carry so much pain within us, or for so long!

The human spirit is like the beauty of the rose. Though at times it may wither, it comes back strong, vibrant, and healthy.

It is not natural for the human body to age and to deteriorate as it does. Our bodies were not designed for this. They were designed to give us long life, robust health, equanimity of mind, and calmness of emotions. We have created the very conditions that erode physical, mental, and emotional health. No one else has created the problems that the majority of the world's population finds itself experiencing.

The diseases that are a scourge upon our planet are the result of our actions and emotions. The many modern plagues that beset us are the result of a planet that has gone out of balance. This lack of balance is due to the intervention and the degradation of our lands. We have stripped bare many acres of prime land, denuding them of nutrition and yet simultaneously setting up the environment for an imbalance of microbes, animals, and plants to exist, thus creating the scenario where ultimately the ecology of our planet is greatly distressed.

As we observe Mother Nature's attempts to rectify the imbalance we have created, please note that the very conditions we find our bodies in are mirroring those of Mother Earth. She is endeavoring to correct the destruction and degradation that has been ongoing, especially so in the last few hundred years of human time. Mother Earth too is like the beauty of the rose. She is now experiencing the winter of her years and is preparing herself for the spring that will emerge. The spring will herald in the new—after there has been a release of the old, after there has been a cleansing of the toxins.

All that we see happening in our natural environment is mirroring what is happening within individuals on our planet. If we were to make some basic changes to our lives, we would find there is no need to suffer from ill health, degenerative conditions, decreased mental functioning, and distressed emotional states as we age. Surely the process of aging is really about the gaining of wisdom, the harnessing and expansion of inner creativity, and the evolvement of greater insight, awareness, and understanding of the meaning of life.

Aging is not about focusing on the little, and, in many instances, not so little ailments. Aging is not about living in fear. It seems that as we age we become more fearful of what is happening in the world around us. We fear for our personal safety. There is great fear around financial insecurity and also around physical health.

Is this what we strive for in our younger years? It seems in many cultures that great emphasis is placed on the accumulation of financial security. This is often in preparation for our older years. It seems the focus for living has become to gain financial security and, accompanying that, there is always the fear of losing it. Should we spend our younger years amassing our fortunes? Given the current lifestyles in developed countries, is there any likelihood that we will have the ability to fully appreciate and enjoy this accumulated wealth? It seems not.

It seems, instead, that no matter how much we amass in terms of financial investments and security, there is never enough. Even if there were, then the fear around losing it and the illnesses generated through emotional stress and mental worry add considerably to the aging process. So it is that when we come to the time of our life when we are most able to enjoy the fruits of our labors, we are instead beset by ailments and conditions that further degenerate our bodies.

It does not have to be like this. We create these conditions. We take on the fears, anxieties, and worries and, through the use of our language and emotions, create what befalls us in our later years. On one level, we know very well that positive thinking creates healthier, happier people. Yet our society, as such, is ingrained with patterns of speech that reinforce negativity and lower self-perceptions.

There are many common expressions that are widely accepted and used within our societies to reinforce the beliefs that life is hard, that aging is inevitable, and that financial struggle is the only way to live. There is a perception that in order to attain a healthy, happy, and safe life one must strive to be in competition, fearful of losing what has been gained. There is an inherent fear that when there is sharing there is also loss.

The human psyche has become so indoctrinated into beliefs about how life must be that it has forgotten that choices can be made—choices in all things, in all ways, and at all times. Nothing is prescribed. The individual creates it through every conscious and subconscious choice.

Where the level of indoctrination is so deep, there is no questioning; there is no examination of what the situation really is. Along with this comes an abrogation of responsibility. The human emotions and mind are very quick to blame others. It is easier to blame an issue, another person, or the system for your ill health or misfortunes. It is much easier to go to someone for a diagnosis and to know that they will take responsibility for healing whatever it is that ails you. That is indeed the preferable option, so it would seem.

Taking full responsibility for all that we do and think requires a huge commitment by the individual. Whenever there is a choice made that is not desired or does not turn out as anticipated, it is often easier to affix the blame elsewhere rather than looking at what has occurred and learning a valuable lesson from it, giving thanks for the opportunity for that learning and then rectifying the situation.

Ironically, in spite of what may appear to be a very gloomy picture that I am painting of the human embodiment, I know that the beauty of the soul still shines through. I know that the soul, like the rose, always blooms when the time is right.

CHAPTER TWO
A Healthy Society?

*"The keenest sorrow is to recognize ourselves
as the sole cause of all our adversities."*
—Sophocles—

"Wouldn't it be wonderful if we could put our fingers on some-one's forehead and say as Jesus did, 'You are now healed,' and that healing would be instantaneous and total?" These words were uttered by one of my many aware clients, who in his own right is a powerful healer.

In a utopian society such a phenomenon would not only be highly desirable, it would also be considered normal. In our current society, however, such a situation would be described as miraculous, if it were to ever occur! There are many seeking the path to awareness and enlighten-ment that also aspire to emulate the miracles of Jesus and other enlight-ened masters. Underlying this aspiration is an inherent belief that in time, with long and diligent seeking, such feats will be achievable.

Upon hearing my client speak longingly of such a possibility, I responded without conscious thought, and my words surprised him as much as they did me. "What you are seeking is an idealization. Instead of a select group of individuals being able to heal to such a degree, we are coming to a time when we will all have the ability to heal our-selves. We look to others to take responsibility for our healing when we, in reality, have this ability within ourselves. To be truly responsible for one's health means that we are then in a position of empowerment when it comes to self-healing."

It has been a few years since that conversation took place, but its clarity remains and has since been replayed within my mind numerous times. As I ponder the message contained in that statement, it is apparent there is much more implied than first appears. The words spoken were clearly guided and as much a message for me as for my client. I wonder, is attaining such a state of empowerment any closer? And, more impor-tantly, are people ready to become fully responsible for their health status? If people are to be truly responsible for their health and well-being, then cul-turally there needs to be a major shift in perception and attitude.

If a time is ever to be reached when all people truly have the ability to self-heal, then a critical step towards achieving this state is acknowl-edging a sense of accountability for creating what has occurred. From there it becomes an individual responsibility to generate the conditions for self-healing to occur and ensure that the best and most relevant healing modalities are applied when appropriate.

At this stage it may seem that what I'm suggesting sounds impossible, especially as societal conditioning and beliefs hold that the mechanisms of the body are too complex for the ordinary person to understand. It is accepted that it is in the public's best interests to leave health matters to the experts. Basically, a system of disempowerment has insidiously been promoted and actively encouraged by both the medical fraternity and pharmaceutical corporations. This has resulted in the gradual diminishing of individual responsibility and ownership of health status.

Health programs focus on illness treatment, not wellness maintenance. Curative medicine predominates. Health funding is given to finding cures, usually at great cost, instead of promoting preventive medicine. Several years ago I remember hearing someone say that in China doctors are remunerated according to the good health of their patients, and that sick patients resulted in low remuneration and status of the doctor within the community!

Realistically, the current system of health care will continue as is until real impetus for change (and improvement) occurs. This will only happen when individuals actively begin to question their medical diagnoses and treatments, instead of meekly accepting what is told to them, and from there taking full responsibility and ownership of the healing process rather than unquestioningly complying with someone else's directives.

Supposing right now you were asked how well you actually feel, what would be your honest response? Do you have sufficient energy for each and every day? Or do you believe it is normal to feel tired, anxious, and to have constant aches and pains in your body? Most people I encounter can list a few symptoms, often minor but annoying, of general discomfort within their bodies. In some instances there is even acceptance that this is normal. This is because within Western society there is an inherent belief that aging inevitably results in degeneration of the body, its organs, and their functioning, and with that there is resultant decreasing energy levels, physical flexibility, and feelings of well-being.

As Western medicine operates on a curative model, most people will generally make a visit to their family doctor a priority only when they do not feel well. For others, it may involve a visit to a natural therapies practitioner, such as chiropractor, naturopath, or acupuncturist. The general response from people when not feeling well is to seek advice, healing, and support from an expert—someone trained in diagnosing and healing whatever the problem or condition may be.

It is normal when experiencing a health problem to seek immediate resolution. Visiting a doctor generally results in the taking of prescription drugs, resting, following prescribed exercises, and sometimes undergoing a surgical procedure. These are common remedies for the great numbers of physical symptoms manifesting within individuals. I have found that focusing attention on physical conditions, however, is only one facet of the total healing process.

The metaphysical meaning of illness, including the link between emotions and health, is nowadays often explored and is gradually gaining acceptance by the general public. Since Louise Hay's early work on the metaphysical meaning of illness, there has been a wealth of research, articles, and books available on the body, mind, and spirit connection.[1] A quick browse through any bookstore usually reveals a quantity of books on "how to" make changes, improve and achieve lasting good health, to have limitless vitality and enhanced wellness, and so on.

Over the years I have seen countless clients experiencing a vast range of conditions involving an extensive range of physical, mental, and emotional discomfort and pain. However, there have been occasions, far too numerous to count, when I have felt helpless and inadequate with the level of my professional ministrations. This is not because of inherent feelings of incompetence or inadequacy. My suspicion is that most healing practitioners will admit to similar feelings in many instances.

The reason for this feeling of inadequacy is that there are often a myriad of symptoms manifesting within the individual seeking healing. Many of these symptoms are deeply emotional and require far more

---

1. Louise Hay. *You Can Heal Yourself*, Hay House, Inc., 1984.

time than I, or any other professional, can possibly give in the course of one or several sessions. It seems as though much of what occurs in healing is often merely a Band-Aid approach, treating the symptoms or obvious pain but not necessarily healing the real cause of ill health. Because of this, no sooner is the healing of one condition facilitated than something else is likely to manifest elsewhere in some other form. A great deal of my work as a healing arts practitioner has been to assist people to come to a greater understanding of how emotions and the mind influence and affect general health and well-being. Many other healing practitioners also adopt and follow similar principles in their work.

It has occurred to me, time and again, that there has to be more to healing than what has been taught, learned, and practiced. Surely there must be some means of ensuring excellent health at all times. After all, this is a given birthright. Most babies are born in a healthy state, as everything within the body is usually in perfect working order at birth. Whatever happens to that healthy body? What causes the body to become increasingly susceptible to illness and poor health? Most importantly of all, what are the conditions creating the general belief that deteriorating health and illness are inevitable and natural? Why, as aging occurs, is it accepted knowledge that either heart disease, cancer, arthritis, or some other dreaded condition will invariably strike? Surely you have the right to expect your body to perform superbly right up until it is time to depart this life.

Given the continuing expansion of knowledge and technology over the last one hundred years, shouldn't there be greater health benefits and improvements on every level? It could be expected that with corresponding changes in diet and lifestyle and advances in medicine, trends should strongly indicate an improvement in general health statistics.

Yet, this is not necessarily the case. Cancers continue proliferating among the general population, with new and unusual cancers on the increase. Heart disease is still considered a major disease despite early detection, intervention, and strategic rehabilitation. The incidence of diabetes is increasing. Fibromyalgia, chronic fatigue, and depression have become commonplace in recent years and could be considered to be in almost epidemic proportions in our Western society. Menopause, which was once a naturally occurring cycle experienced by women, is now considered to be another disease or condition that requires extensive research, testing, and medicating. The list goes on and on. There are numerous newly identified conditions and illnesses that devour millions of dollars annually in extensive research and testing.

It should be noted that the three main causes of death in industrialized countries are heart disease, cancer, and iatrogenic deaths. "Iatrogenic" means caused by medical treatment. In the United States alone, research figures indicate that 225,000 deaths occur annually due to unnecessary surgery, medication errors, miscellaneous errors in hospitals, infections in hospitals, and negative effects of drugs. It has also been suggested that this figure of 225,000 is somewhat conservative.[2]

A recent article reported that in 2003, health care spending reached $1.6 trillion in the United States.[3] The article also states, "We actually cause more illness through medical technology, diagnostic testing, overuse of medical and surgical procedures and overuse of pharmaceutical drugs. The huge disservice of this therapeutic strategy is the result of little effort or money being appropriated for preventing disease." This article, complex in its research data, also indicates strongly that the rate of iatrogenic deaths is far greater than previously believed. By projecting the available research statistics over a ten-year span, the figure of 7.8 million iatrogenic deaths is postulated. This figure is far "more than all the casualties from wars that America has fought in its entire history."

The reality is that twentieth-century health conditions continue unabated regardless of the amount of money spent in research, development, medication, and eradication programs. The health status of the general population is as precarious now as it ever has been. This is in spite of the development of wonder drugs such as antibiotics, better standards of personal and public hygiene, and vast improvements in living standards in the last hundred years or so. Isn't it time to stop and seriously question whether what we are doing is actually working?

---

2. Phillip Day. *Health Wars*, Credence Publications, 2001.

3. Carolyn Dean, MD ND, Martin Feldman, MD, Gary Null, PhD, and Debora Rasio, MD. "Death By Medicine," *Nexus New Times* 11, no. 5. Refer to website: www.nutritioninstituteofamerica.org.

Ours is an era in which scientific analysis and reasoning predominate. If something can be proved and validated, it is accepted as a scientific truth. Scientific inquiry always follows a structured process. There is the initial hypothesis or theory put forward. In order to prove it, logical steps are then adhered to in observation and testing situations. A control group or study is generally included as a means of ensuring validation. This is the process followed by medical and scientific researchers which invariably results in a vast array of new products (medications) being made available for public consumption as an aid to achieving health improvement or hinting at possible cures for a range of illnesses.

However, it has to be obvious to anyone that our way of dealing with health issues is not effective. Escalating health costs are affecting the whole of society. Health insurance in Western countries is becoming increasingly expensive. In fact, it is becoming so expensive that it is rapidly becoming unaffordable. Health statistics may indicate improvement in some conditions and diseases, but overall it seems that more and more people are at greater risk of developing ill health or a serious health condition during their life. Ill health is rapidly becoming an acceptable state of being for a significant portion of the population in this country!

My contention is that real and lasting healing is not being achieved because attention is not focused in the right direction or in all possible directions. Scientific research and development deals with the physiological and anatomical aspects (data has to be measurable and validated) and is generally limited to facilitating healing of the physical body. However, the figures quoted previously, demonstrating the high rate of iatrogenic deaths, are an indication that this methodology isn't achieving promising results!

The metaphysical approach, dealing with emotional and mental states, is a healing modality that is gaining acceptance by the general public and is often used in conjunction with standard medical treatments. In recent years the benefits of spiritual healing, whether through religious faith or spiritual convictions, has been acknowledged as being a valid form of healing. The healing power of meditation and prayer has been validated in research studies.[4]

Irrespective of the type of healing approach undertaken, in most instances the patient tends to rely on the expertise and experience of someone else. Societal conditioning and health models are constructed in such a manner that trusting other people to know what is best for us has become the modus operandi for the population in general. With this there is also the possibility of a codependency situation arising, as the patient may come to rely heavily on the skills of the practitioner to cure whatever ailment is being treated. However, the corollary of this is that it has become all too easy to abdicate self-responsibility for our health. In looking to others to prescribe quick fixes and painless solutions to health issues, complacency sets in and individual learning and problem solving skills diminish.

Realistically, healing is a gradual process. Anyone who has suffered the frustration of a broken limb or heart attack can assure you there is no quick fix for this type of healing. It is the same for practically every other illness or health-related condition. Ill health does not occur overnight; rather, it occurs stealthily over time and often without obvious initial warning signs. For healing to be beneficial and lasting, a process involving indeterminate time, depending upon conditions of ill health, takes place as the body restores itself to a state of homeostasis.

In the following chapters I will be proposing an unorthodox and possibly different perspective on how the body functions and heals. I ask that you keep an open mind and suspend judgment because it is very likely your beliefs will be challenged. From what I share, you will be able to gain a basic understanding of how healing works on a much broader basis.

By making some straightforward changes to your lifestyle, you will be able to create a healthy and balanced body, one that will remain

---

4. Joan Budilovsky and Eve Adamson. *The Complete Idiot's Guide to Meditation*, Alpha, 2003., Eric Harrison. *Teach Yourself to Meditate in 10 Simple Lessons*, Ulysses Press, 2000, Michael Levin. *Meditation: Path to the Deepest Self*, OK Publishing, Inc., 2002., www.tm.org/research/home. html, www.hno.harvard.edu/gazette/2002/04.18/09-tummo.html, www.newscientist.com/article.ns?id=dn8317

healthy for as long as you consciously choose. Strategies and visualization exercises are also included throughout the book. In implementing the suggested changes, know that you will be taking charge of your own health status. You will come to know and view your body intimately and certainly in a way not experienced before.

My intention in sharing the information in this book is to create awareness so that you can make empowered and conscious health-related decisions for your highest good. Finally, how do I know that what I'm sharing works? Because I apply the principles in my life consciously and consistently. My health has never been better, and it has been that way for some years now in spite of the fact that I'm in my mid-fifties, which is the time of life when one supposedly begins succumbing to many degenerative conditions and diseases.

As you read and come to understand the basis of the information, you too will come to see your potential for creating improvements in all areas of your life. Having good health and well-being is a choice that is available to all. It is how you live and view your life that ultimately makes all the difference.

CHAPTER THREE
Understanding the Body

"Not everything that counts can be counted
and not everything that can be counted counts."
—Albert Einstein—

Over the last hundred years or more scientific research has delved deeper to uncover more and more about the amazingly complex piece of machinery that is the human body. There is no denying that scientifically and medically there have been incredible discoveries about the structure and functioning of the physical body, and, with that, there have been dramatic improvements in testing, diagnosis and surgery procedures. Allopathic, or Western, medicine predominates in our society. Allopathic medicine focuses on the physical body; it focuses on what can be seen, whether with the naked eye or under a microscope. It is premised on scientific theory and research and is the yardstick by which individuals gauge their well-being.

Not all cultures, however, advocate or support the allopathic model. Ancient texts and teachings show we are more than a physical body. Traditional Chinese and Indian medicines, which are holistically based, have been used successfully for thousands of years and were established long before allopathic medicine became fashionable. It must also be remembered that indigenous cultures throughout the world have used plant medicine successfully for thousands of years. Allopathic medicine could realistically be viewed as the new kid on the block when placed within the larger context of all medicines that have been developed and adopted. Being the latest model does not necessarily mean it is superior nor is it necessarily likely to supersede earlier medical models.

Allopathic medicine focuses primarily on the treatment of the physical body and generally does not acknowledge that we are more than a physical body when it comes to treating ailments. The reason for this is that allopathic theory presumes pathogen states are present when ill health occurs, and so treatment is commonly based on medication and surgical procedures.

Being holistic models, both traditional Chinese medicine and ancient Indian knowledge and practices acknowledge the energy field that is part of the body. This energy field is part of and also surrounds the physical body. In Chinese medicine this energy is known as *Ch'I*. It is a vital energy containing two opposite forces, yin and yang. When these opposing forces are balanced, the body is in a state of health and, when out of balance, a state of dis-ease is the result—dis-ease meaning lack of ease or comfort. Ancient Indian teachings refer extensively to *prana*, which is otherwise known as universal life energy. Prana includes spiritual breath or light energy and is vital to healthy bodily functioning. Yoga practitioners are well aware of the importance of correct breathing techniques in maintaining suppleness and vitality with the spiritual breath.

Eastern philosophies and teachings have successfully made their way into Western culture, especially since the 1960s and are now being integrated in countless ways into health care practices. This has provided the general population with a clear opportunity to learn about other medical models, spiritual practices, and beliefs. Societally, this has resulted in a greater diversity of choices.

Many holistic teachers and practitioners have taught and written about the different bodies the individual has, including information as to the importance of these bodies to overall health and well-being. There are seven such bodies, each having a specific function. The first is the physical-etheric body, which comprises the dense physical body. Close to the physical body are the astral and mental bodies. Further out are four higher bodies, often referred to as the intuitional, atmic, monadic, and divine planes.[5] In the extensive literature that is available, different words have been used as descriptors of definition and function, but their meaning and intent are much the same. For the purposes of this book, I am taking the liberty of simplifying explanations that could easily fill another book. It is my intention to provide a broad overview in order that later descriptions and explanations have an identifiable context.

The work of medical intuitives, including Barbara Brennan and Dr. Carolyn Myss, has been influential in the lives of many people in Western cultures. Their books and teachings have taken a great deal from Eastern perspectives on how the body is formed and how it functions. They have demonstrated that it is as important to have awareness of and care for your energy field as it is your physical body. Dr. Carolyn Myss and others have demonstrated the vital role performed by the seven chakras, or energy centers, in the body that record and

---

5. Torkom Saraydarian. *New Dimensions in Healing*, T.S.G. Publishing Foundation, 1992.

store information about your emotions, experiences, and beliefs.[6] These teachings stress the importance of good management of the chakras, which in turn leads to balance and well-being in daily life.

In her books, *Hands of Light* and *Emerging Light*, Barbara Brennan illustrates and explains clearly how the chakras and the energy field operate. She has identified seven layers within the energy field that surrounds the body, with each layer having a distinct purpose. These layers are briefly summarized below. In order to understand this concept more easily, imagine your physical body standing erect and being enveloped by these invisible layers extending outward.

- The first layer, closest to the physical body, is associated with physical functioning and sensation.

- The emotional body is stored in the second layer. It is often easy to see people's emotions for they are stored so close to the physical body.

- Mental or cognitive processing is located in the third layer.

- How you relate to love, including all forms of love—relationships, familial, and humanitarian—is stored in the fourth layer.

- The fifth layer is associated with speaking, listening, and taking responsibility for your thoughts and actions.

- The sixth layer is about celestial love and extends beyond love for humanity. It relates to a belief in something bigger, that is, God, the Source, Creator, or whatever name you ascribe to this concept.

- Finally, the seventh layer relates to the higher mind and is about connecting with a spiritual source, which integrates with and is integral to your physical reality.

It is interesting to note that the functioning of these seven energy layers correlates closely to the seven core chakras of the human body. A chakra is a vortex of energy that functions or spins within the energy layers discussed above and is critical to your life force. C.W. Leadbeater

---

6.   Carolyn Myss. *Energetics of Healing,* two tape videocassette.

published the definitive work on chakras in 1927.[7] Since then, there has been substantial research and information made available on working with and creating healthy chakras.

- The first chakra is the root chakra, which is located at the base of the spine. This chakra stores beliefs about society and culture and correlates to the first layer of the energy field.

- The sacral chakra, or second chakra, is found just below the navel. This energy vortex stores beliefs around sexuality, power, business, and how you perceive other people and is connected to the second layer—emotions—in the energy field.

- The solar plexus houses the third chakra, which relates to how individuals view themselves and their feelings about life and people in general. This corresponds to the third layer in the energy field, that of mental or cognitive functioning.

- The heart center is the fourth chakra and is located mid-chest. It is closely connected to how you love on an unconditional basis.

- The fifth chakra is located in the throat area and indicates an ability to speak your spiritual truth. It is closely aligned to the fifth layer.

- The sixth chakra is found between the eyebrows and is commonly referred to as the "third eye." It accesses other dimensions and realms, and it is through this third eye that clairvoyance is said to occur. This chakra is about spiritual awareness and is linked to the sixth layer, which is about celestial love.

- The seventh and final chakra is located on the crown of the head and is the connection to a divine source. Similarly, the seventh layer is about connecting with a higher source.

Understanding the energy field, its layers, and the chakra system is important for medical intuitives who work with the energy centers and layers. Medical intuitives are able to see (using the third eye) ill health within the energy field. In this way they are able to assist the individual

---

7. C. W. Leadbeater. *The Chakras,* Theosophical Publishing House, 1927.

and, in some instances, allopathic medical professionals with diagnosis and the healing process.

If the energy field is part of you, how can you ascertain exactly what is stored in the physical body and what is stored within the invisible energy field? This is purely a rhetorical question, for there can be no separating the physical from the energetic. In lay terms, I prefer to say that an energy field surrounds the physical body. The reality, though, is that your physical body is actually an integral and interconnected part of the whole energy field.

All energy vibrates, though not necessarily at the same frequency. This means, for example, that matter that is more dense or solid vibrates at a lower frequency. Energy of a higher frequency is not discernible to the ordinary eye. Examples of these include microwaves, electromagnetic waves, and the human energy field. The physical body is mostly dense energy, and the surrounding energy layers become lighter and finer the further away they are from the body. Similarly, the further away the energy layers are the higher the vibrational frequency becomes. Each individual energy field connects with universal energy, which is everywhere. The nothingness that is felt and seen is energy. The solid physical reality of the world is surrounded and filled with a "fluid world of radiating energy, constantly moving, constantly changing like the sea."[8]

This means that whatever is experienced in life is first felt in the outer energy field. Everything is filtered through the energy field in order to be felt and received on a physical level. A clear example of this occurs when you first meet someone and have an immediate and instinctual sense of his or her character and personality. Your energy field connects with theirs and from that you glean information about them. All this happens rapidly and intuitively, but nevertheless you are able to ascertain a great deal about someone or something because of what occurs in the energy field.

It cannot be stressed too strongly that the energy field is vitally important to your health and well-being. Any imbalance or distortion

---

8. Barbara Ann **Brennan**. *Hands of Light*, Bantam Books, 1988.

in the energy field will ultimately manifest as dis-ease or illness in the physical body. When all layers of the energy field are strong and balanced, a healthy physical body is evident.

In Western societies it is commonly accepted that the concept of self exists within the physical body. Because of this, it is easy to overlook the importance of recognizing and acknowledging that the human body is more than its physical state. When focus and interest is placed exclusively on the physical body, you neglect a large part of who you really are. When concentrating solely on your physicality, you either energize or drain your physical body with thoughts and emotions.

This can be clearly explained using a simple analogy. Imagine you have recently purchased a new home. If all your time, energy, and money go into ensuring the furnishings in your home are exquisite and perfect but you ignore the maintenance required to keep the house functioning, you will most likely end up with some serious problems. In time, the outside might need painting. The plumbing could fail. The garden would be neglected, giving an unkempt appearance. Overall, there would be an imbalance between the outer and inner, which ultimately would create greater problems, anxiety, and cost to you, the homeowner.

It is the same with your body. When one aspect (physical) of the body receives all your attention and other aspects (layers of the energy field) are excluded, health problems result. It does not happen suddenly. Rather, it is a slow and steady process. Yet when ill health strikes, it is a common reaction to question how this could have happened. The reason for unexpected ill health is often blamed on something tangible, such as recent events or even other people! This is because Western cultures are imbued with the belief that what can be seen, felt, touched, smelled, or heard is the only reality due to their tangibility. It is often difficult to accept that there is more to reality than what medicine and science have taught.

Ironically, I've observed that generally people expend more energy in ensuring their cars function optimally than on their wellness. Time is devoted to getting to know your car, finding out what gas and oils are most appropriate, becoming familiar with or tuning into its performance, and knowing when maintenance is required. This means you maximize your car's reliability and performance, as well as reducing the likelihood of an unexpected breakdown or malfunction. I believe that the ability to be equally "in tune" with the workings of the body is inherent within each and every one of us! Years ago when I studied basic computing processes, I remember clearly being told, "Garbage in, garbage out." The same principle applies to the human body.

When the body is valued as a sacred vessel, you are more likely to treat it with respect and ensure that only premium-quality breath, thoughts, foods, and so on are ever given to it. The human body has been genetically engineered and designed to last well beyond the current anticipated lifespan. It is an incredibly beautiful and complex piece of machinery. It serves you well on all levels—physical, mental, emotional, and spiritual. Each level is part of you and deserves optimum care.

For the purposes of this book, I will refer mainly to the four levels mentioned above. It is for ease of explanation and hopefully will provide a point of reference and understanding, and in no way is intended to diminish the importance of the chakra and energy layer systems. An outline of what each level means and its interconnectedness with the seven chakras and layers of the energy field follows:

- The physical level refers to all aspects of the physical body, its maintenance, and its functioning. The physical body is the most familiar. It is what is reflected back whenever you look in the mirror. The base chakra and first layer are connected to the physical level.

- The mental level refers to mind states and cognitive and intellectual functioning. This level connects with the third chakra and the third layer of the energy field.

- The emotional level relates to both human emotional responses, which are situated in the second chakra and energy layer, as well as to humanitarian love and spiritual unconditional love. These are found in the heart center (fourth chakra).

- The spiritual level and awareness are found in the throat, third eye and crown chakras, or fifth to seventh layers of the energy field. Additionally, there is an overlap with the emotional level, as unconditional love is spiritually based.

Balance is the keyword that underpins everything in life. When the physical, mental, emotional, and spiritual levels are in balance, there is a resultant increase in wellness and vitality. How is it possible to achieve balance on all levels? This requires some basic knowledge of how the levels function and how to best nourish and heal them. It requires putting into practice some straightforward and effective changes into daily life. It requires being aware and mindful of what is negative or harmful and what is positive and creative. Being balanced is not something that happens after participating in a six, ten, or twelve-week program. It requires continual awareness and adjustment because life itself is fraught with challenges, unexpected surprises, and countless stresses.

In gaining an understanding of how energy works, you will find that coming to a state of balance becomes easier. An important lesson I've learned in life is that if you don't know which questions to ask you won't always receive the information you're seeking. It is with this in mind that strategies have been included throughout this book to assist you to come to greater awareness of energy, how your body works energetically, and also how to implement changes to create the awareness and balance you are seeking. In addition, visualization exercises are also included. This is to assist your manifesting abilities, to offer a means of quieting the mind, and to support your journey into expanded awareness.

CHAPTER FOUR

Everything is Energy

"We rarely hear the inward music,
but we're all dancing to it nevertheless."
—Maulana Jalalu'ddin Rumi—

There is no doubt that the study of energy has a predominant place in the rapidly expanding field of quantum physics, quantum mechanics, and technology. In scientific terms, energy can mean many things. It may refer to the field of quantum physics or to the capacity of matter to do work. The work of Tesla, Einstein, Max Planck, and others has unmasked many of the mysteries surrounding this invisible, yet powerful, force. These are only a few of the many scientists who have explored the nature of matter and interconnectedness. To date scientists have been able to extensively study and analyze the human energy field.

As research and technology expand and greater awareness within populations occurs, the understanding that the human body consists of more than mere physical form is becoming gradually acknowledged. With that comes acceptance of the permanent presence of an energy field, comprising several layers, around the physical body. Quantum physics teaches that nothing is random, that there is structure even amid chaos. So it is with the energy field that is the body. The physical cannot be separated from the nonphysical. The two are integrated, inseparable, interconnected, and essential for human functioning in every respect.

In spiritual and New Age terminology, energy is frequently used to describe an unseen force, though often it is viewed as something that is not clearly quantifiable or definable. For example, a regular comment expressed by individuals is that the vibes, or energies, around a place or person are good. This means that individual, in some manner, feels comfortable being in a particular environment or with a certain person. Or, of course, the opposite may also be true. It is also possible to be in places or with people where the energies feel heavy, scattered, or dark. As was mentioned in the previous chapter, Eastern tradition is steeped in energy consciousness. Many traditional teachings and practices refer to this energy force. There is a vast amount of information available, whether one is interested in bodywork, Buddhism, or theosophy, to name but a few.

Each person has a unique energy field that constantly changes due to what is happening in life and through his or her interaction with others. Kirlian photography shows the energy emanating from an individual's hands. Aura readings are common nowadays and always create interest for the individual wanting to see what actually surrounds his or her body.

Deepak Chopra, author of many books on healing and spiritual matters, often refers to energy in terms of quantum physics to explain how the human form is composed and how it functions. In his book, *How to Know God,* Chopra explores the concept of the mind and in doing so suggests that the mind and brain are not necessarily the same thing, though there is a strong connection between the two.[9] It is proposed, instead, that the mind is an invisible energy field that experiences whatever happens, and this is then recorded in the brain for retention.

It is said that energy is the basis of all life. Years ago, high school science classes taught cellular structure, whether in solid, liquid, or gaseous composition, as consisting of a nucleus around which atoms move in a circular or oval rotation. In between the nucleus and atoms there was always space. That space was then referred to as "space." Science now acknowledges that this space is not empty. It is filled with energy. In fact, there is no such thing as empty space. For example, when one item is removed from a habitat or environment, energy moves in to fill the space. Likewise, it takes energy to move energy. This is the basis upon which energy healing works.

In order to best explain my understanding of how energy works in the human body, I will describe as simply as possible how my awareness occurred and then will outline the implication this energy model holds for the healing process. My understanding did not come about suddenly, as if in a revelation. Rather, it was a slow and steady process of learning that led me to the information I am now ready to share.

In order to place this information into a structured context, it is necessary to outline some of my background and the experiences that led to the acquisition of this knowledge. It was during the early '90s when my interest in esoteric principles and studies suddenly escalated. This involved reading about such matters, undertaking a process of self-healing that has taken many years, engaging in regular meditation, as well as opening up and learning to trust my sixth sense, or intuitive

---

9.   Deepak Chopra. *How To Know God*, Rider Books, 2000.

knowing. During this time there was also the discovery of a gift I had inherited from my great-grandmother, who was a natural healer. My father shared stories of how she would place her hands on a person and their pain would disappear. Eventually I was guided to Reiki and thought this was how my gift of healing abilities would be used. It was, but only for a while. It seems that life is a journey and as I took each new step, often with hesitation, I found myself thinking, "This is it!" only to realize eventually that it was merely one small step out of many still to be taken.

Reiki and spiritual healing were two modalities that I used with success, and they were a large part of my learning. By the late '90s my full-time employment was in the area of bodywork, including energy work. I was also working strongly with my intuition, having learned that whenever my intuition was ignored and logic was applied that outcomes were usually disastrous. During this period in the '90s I also became aware of other energy beings or spirits, invisible to the naked eye, around me. This became a common occurrence, especially when working in my healing room or meditating. Even though they could not be seen with my naked eye, their presence was strongly sensed. Occasionally I was privileged to see them through my third eye, and this occurred generally during daily meditations. Over time, telepathic communication was established with them.

Initially there was hesitation and skepticism on my part regarding practically everything I was told. My response was to question consistently and to ask for proof. I was not satisfied with only hearing and therefore demanded demonstrable outcomes. And I got them, time and time again. It was a tedious process but having been brought up with a strong adherence to the principles of scientific study, I certainly wasn't about to be duped. Needless to say, I learned to trust my friends from other dimensions and the knowledge they imparted. Their guidance and assistance in my healing room and in countless other aspects of life became, and continue to be, invaluable.

In early 2000, there was a visitation in my healing room from energy beings I had not encountered previously. By this stage I had become adept at recognizing the vibrational energy signature of certain beings and immediately felt that these new visitors emanated extremely high energies. It must be mentioned that my awareness to sensing or feeling energies is due to extensive and deep spiritual experiences. When I questioned their presence in my room, they indicated that they had come to teach me, if I was willing. My agreement was immediately forthcoming. This was not something I had consciously requested during my meditation sessions, yet on an instinctual level it felt completely right and appropriate. On a rational level, my interest in learning was still strong. I was always eager to acquire new skills and knowledge. These energy beings shared that they would teach me about healing, the human body, energy, and other relevant topics. My learning commenced then and still continues.

The mind has an incredible capacity to learn vast amounts of information providing the individual is receptive and willing to have old beliefs updated. It is easy to learn that the world is flat and to hold that as a truth. In much the same way, as an example, it was once believed that the Earth was the center of our galaxy. That belief was held by society for a long time and was shattered by the work of Copernicus who stated with absolute certainty that the sun held that honored position. Interestingly, he only shared this knowledge with the wider society as his life was nearing its end. Maybe it was because he no longer feared reprisals from authority figures for daring to prove their knowledge to be wrong!

When you are ready to let go of old truths, to explore the world and your perception of reality, with no limitations, then you also have to be willing to take that next step into the unknown. It is healthy to consciously open your mind and heart to other ways of perceiving and being. When doing this, it is usually necessary to leave behind some long-held beliefs and ways of living. Consequently, reality may change dramatically and permanently as a result of taking such a step. However, the sense of adventure and curiosity is strong in most people. It certainly is in me, and in time what I've learned will be superseded by something else. This will occur when there is acceptance and readiness to integrate whatever new learning is appropriate and relevant.

So it was that my new learning began in earnest from early 2000. I was asked by these energy beings to stop reading books and articles and to not attend any further workshops, as they would be my teachers. Without hesitation I accepted their request. The reason for this was so that my hearing and understanding would be clear and without interference or confusion, which would happen if I were to access other, human-interpreted, sources of information.

On reflection, the information presented by them was structured and paced, though there were times when I was in a hurry to learn more. Maybe there was a lesson in patience being taught! The healing abilities I had been gifted with changed gradually and still continue to change. I saw different things within people's energy fields and was shown how to balance and realign energies so that the body could heal itself. I was shown how illness manifests and how we unwittingly contribute to and create the very illnesses and conditions we seek healing for.

Their teaching occurred in my healing room, during daily meditations, through automatic writing, channeling, and also during lucid dreams. At this time I already had an understanding of the chakra system as well as the aura. It was from their teaching that I came to view the aura as an emanating energy that reveals what is happening within emotions and thoughts at any one time. The aura and energy field are interlinked, with the energies of the aura impinging on what occurs within the energy field. The energy field is distinctly different. It can be viewed as both a receiver and transmitter of universal energy.

In books, the energy field is generally portrayed as layers of light radiating outward from the physical body. (Refer to figure 1 at the end of the chapter.) However, I have been shown the energy field somewhat differently to how it is generally depicted. My sense is that what has been shown is the actual structure, or breakdown into finer detail, of the energy field that is currently depicted in available literature.

This is what I have been shown clearly many times and is actually how the energy field is structured and operates. Imagine a sheet of graph paper. It consists of parallel grid lines running in a north-south direction and intersecting parallel lines running in an east-west direction. Now imagine this sheet of graph paper in an upright position. Behind and in front of it are many other sheets of similar graph paper in line. The space between the sheets is not empty. There are more lines between the sheets. These lines intersect diagonally and horizontally, joining the many sheets of graph paper together. (Refer to figure 2 at the end of the chapter.) The grid lines are very fine, spun like silken thread. Along these grid lines microscopic golden balls of energy whiz in all directions. (Refer to figure 3 at the end of the chapter.) The golden balls of energy are the *Ch'I* or *Prana* that were mentioned in an earlier chapter. It is these fine silken threads with the golden balls of energy moving at an incredibly rapid rate that form the whole web of the energy field, including the physical body.

Now imagine a finely woven and intricate spider's web. This too is another web of life, as the web is the spider's home and sustains its quest for food and nourishment. When a spider's web is partially or fully destroyed, the spider either has to undertake repairs or build a new web. Whatever is left has been changed from its original structure and composition. It is damaged in some way and cannot be used as it was. Fortunately for the spider, it has the ability to weave a new web and so is not left without means of sustaining itself.

The human energy field, or web, also experiences damage in many ways and on an almost continual basis. Many times I have seen this web of energy grids distorted, fractured, compacted, distended, and out of alignment. (Refer to figures 4, 5, and 6 at the end of the chapter.) The analogy I often use to describe this is what happens to an exquisitely hand-knitted woolen sweater that is washed in hot water. Prior to the washing, the wool is clearly patterned, its structure and shape perfectly formed. However, after washing the wool fibers become compacted, distorted, and misshapen.

This is precisely what happens to our energy field over time because the world is filled with toxins. We cannot escape them. Exposure to toxins is unavoidable in twenty-first century living. Toxins are found in foods and in the environment. Emotions and thoughts are often toxic. All stress and toxins impact on our susceptible energy field in ways that are still not fully understood. Their impact is undoubtedly damaging, as our energy webs are so finely tuned and highly sensitive, much like the spider's web! Eventually, after prolonged periods of exposure to stress and toxins, the energy field ends up being out of balance, the energies become misaligned and weakened (Refer to figure 8 at the end of the chapter.) resulting in a state of dis-ease, discomfort, or ill health. It is common for the energy field to hold emotional and other trauma blockages, and an example of this is shown in figure 7 at the end of the chapter.

What this tells me is that in some way the energy field is a living, dynamic structure. It is highly responsive to whatever occurs within and around it. The energy field appears to have consciousness. It seems to be aware of what is both beneficial and harmful, and then responds accordingly. As a dynamic structure there is also scope for its growth and expansion because it obviously never remains in a constant state.

The question now is, how to heal such a damaged energy field? Or, more importantly, what is needed to create and maintain a healthy energy field? There are many aspects involved in rebalancing and realigning the energy field back to a state of homeostasis. These will be covered in later chapters, along with further explanations of how illness manifests and why healing must take place from an outside to inner perspective rather than working solely with the physical body. Real and lasting healing involves working with the whole energetic web, comprised of this intricate grid-like structure. Any other form of healing is merely a Band-Aid, offering temporary treatment.

Feeling Energy

The following exercises will only take a few minutes and are designed so you will connect with and feel energy. If you have not felt energy before, several attempts may be needed. However, please persevere, as having success with these two exercises will then pave the way for being successful with the other exercises provided in this book.

Sit comfortably wherever you choose. Keep your back straight, your legs uncrossed, and your feet on the floor. Rest your arms gently on your lap. Breathe in deeply and slowly. Exhale gently. Repeat this breath cycle a few times.

Now concentrate on totally relaxing your body. Feel your shoulders drop into a relaxed position as you release tension from this area. Continue breathing gently and deeply. With each inhalation, feel the air expand your lungs. With each exhalation, feel tension releasing from every part of your body.

Slowly bring your arms down by the side of your body, feeling them hanging loosely at your side. Your arms and hands are light and airy. All tension has completely washed away.

Focus your attention back to your breath. As you breathe deeply and gently, very slowly bend your elbows and bring both arms up toward your navel. As you continue to raise your arms, gradually bring your hands up near your heart, with your palms facing each other nearly a foot apart. Imagine a ball of empty space between your hands. Hold this position momentarily while maintaining a relaxed state in your arms and hands. Be aware of any sensations circulating throughout your arms and body.

Slowly continue moving your hands closer to one another. A moment will arrive when you feel resistance to the forward movement, as though your hands have encountered an obstacle. Hold both hands still when you encounter that resistance. The distance between your hands may be several inches or more. Once you encounter this space of resistance, it will feel as though you are holding a ball of energy in your hands. You are feeling your energy field as it exists between your hands. Now begin playing with it. Move your hands slowly apart, and then bring them together again until you feel the resistance. Stretch the energy in different directions. Shape and play with the energy, feeling its versatility and subtlety. You may experience a tingling sensation or warmth running through your hands. Make a note of how you are experiencing and feeling this energy.

When you have finished interacting with this energy, bring your arms further apart and back to a comfortable resting position. Inhale and exhale steadily, then gradually bring your consciousness back to the room.

Sensational Stillness

Sit comfortably wherever you choose. Keep your back straight, your legs uncrossed, and your feet on the floor. Rest your arms gently on your lap. Breathe in deeply and slowly. Exhale gently. Inhale, letting the air flow into your chest, gradually around your ribs, and finally into your entire abdomen. Now exhale, first from your abdomen, then your ribs, and finally your chest. Repeat this process slowly, feeling your breath moving throughout your body.

Now relax your body further, let your shoulders drop, and hold your head erect and aligned with your spine. When comfortable, close your eyes and focus on breathing slowly and deeply. As you do this, allow your thoughts to dissolve. Allow yourself a respite from your mind's ceaseless chatter. Feel your breath. Become aware of the stillness within as all thoughts disappear. Feel your breath releasing stored tension with each exhalation.

When your body and mind are in a relaxed state, focus your attention on what you are sensing and feeling. What is happening within and around you? Be aware of any changes or unusual sensations. Do not question them; merely follow them.

Do you feel tingling or sensations of warmth? Are you aware of a pulsing movement, similar to the motion of waves? Are there other unusual movements or feelings occurring? Make a note of what you feel and sense. Whatever subtle sensations you experience are energy. This is how you sense or feel energy. Allow yourself a few minutes of complete relaxation before gradually bringing your awareness back into the room.

When you have fully returned to the room, spend a few minutes reflecting on your experience. Note what you experienced and how it felt. Responses to this exercise depend greatly on the individual.

Fig. 1

The human energy field radiates outwardly with the densest vibration closer to the body, and the very finest a tthe outer edges.

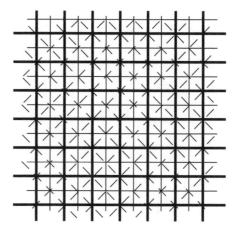

Fig. 2

Energy Grid Structure

This is a three dimensional structure (as a matrix)

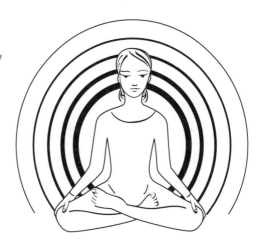

Fig. 3

Side View of Energy Grid

The dots indicate energy in constant motion.

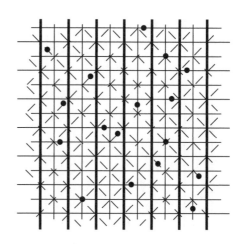

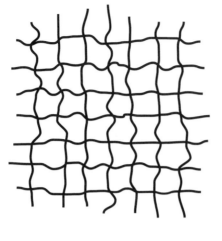

Fig. 4

Distorted Energy Grid

The energy grid no longer resembles a regular matrix. Energy flow becomes erratic and sluggish.

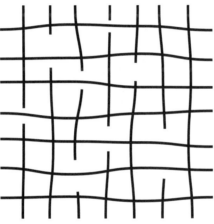

Fig. 5

Fractured Energy Grid

The energy grid has distinct breaks (fractures), which interfere with energy flow.

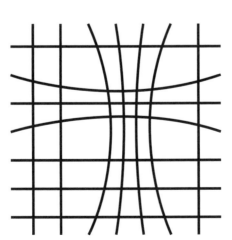

Fig. 6

Compacted Energy Grid

The grid structure compresses, resulting in unevenness. Over time this produces tension in the energy grid.

Fig. 7

Energy Blockage

Accumulated energy is stored, creating a significant blockage to the energy flow.

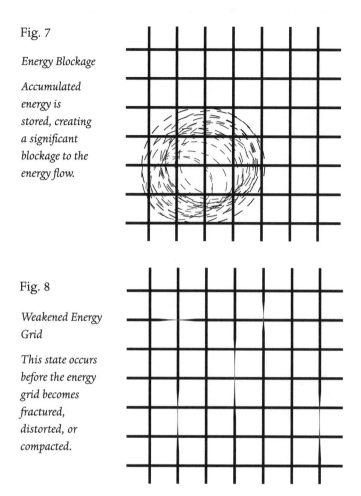

Fig. 8

Weakened Energy Grid

This state occurs before the energy grid becomes fractured, distorted, or compacted.

CHAPTER FIVE
Outside-In
Perspective

"Condemnation without investigation
is the height of ignorance."
—Albert Einstein—

In our culture it is common to seek the services and skills of a doctor when experiencing signs of illness or discomfort. As the study of medicine has become more sophisticated and knowledgeable, a vast array of fitting solutions have evolved to help cure whatever ailments people experience. Usually such solutions relate mainly to healing the physical body, which is where the symptoms of malaise are manifesting. In many situations there is no immediate cure for whatever ails the individual. Often the exact nature of the condition is indeterminate as various symptoms present themselves, thus requiring extensive testing in order to determine the cause of illness.

Time itself is a great healer. Yet this seems to have been mostly forgotten. People in Western cultures are geared to expect immediate results and instant gratification in practically all aspects of life. In this regard there is often the perception that there must be a "quick fix" available for whatever creates pain and discomfort. An example of this is the pain experienced with headaches. Unless the headache is a commonly recurring experience, most people will swallow a couple of tablets (painkillers) to ease the pain. It is only when the headaches continue on a regular basis that there is the likelihood of tests being conducted to see if there is a deeper cause. A headache is basically a symptom, or indication, of something that is not working properly. Treating the symptom with painkillers will not necessarily in any way treat the actual cause of the discomfort. It merely reduces or dulls the symptom, which happens to be the headache itself.

Not all pain is physical, and it is common to experience spiritual, emotional, or mental distress. Such pain is real, and finding the appropriate treatment is not always an easy or straightforward task. In these situations, the consumer is faced with a wider range of practitioners to choose from. The services of analysts and therapists are widely sought after, especially when it comes to emotional issues around relationships and other life issues. For such situations the skills of allopathic practitioners are also commonly sought. In some situations medication is prescribed to help the individual come to a state of calmness in order to better be able to cope with the stresses of life. For example, depression is now a commonly diagnosed condition, with many people prescribed antidepressant tablets. Again, the solution is focused on medicating the physical body where the symptoms have manifested.

According to Dean et al., a "whole generation of antidepressant users has resulted from young people growing up on Ritalin. Medicating youth and modifying their emotions must have some impact on how they learn to deal with their feelings. They learn to equate coping with drugs and not with their inner resources."[10] Research now is indicating a link between antidepressant consumption and increasing risk of suicidal behavior, especially among children and teenagers.[11]

Current trends, however, point to a growing awareness and acceptance among the public that other options are readily available for achieving healing. A growth industry is springing up in all Western countries as holistic practitioners, adopting Eastern philosophies and practices, integrate them into a variety of modalities. These modalities offer a holistic perspective. The patient seeking help for headaches may, instead of taking pain-reducing tablets, opt for a series of acupuncture or flower essence treatments. Similarly, the patient suffering emotional pain due to life stresses may choose to have massage treatments and aromatherapy in addition to visiting a therapist regularly.

Nowadays, treatment options available to the general public are vastly increased. The most difficult choice confronting the consumer is often to know which modality will be most beneficial. What works for one person's condition may not necessarily be the most appropriate for another. Different people experiencing symptoms of regular headaches, for example, may have entirely different causes for those headaches. Acupuncture treatments may provide relief for one person; for another it may be chiropractic adjustments, and for a third person several Reiki sessions may be the solution. It literally depends on what is actually occurring within the unique biochemistry and physiology of each individual. Needless to say, on an energetic level it also depends largely on

10. Carolyn Dean, MD ND, Martin Feldman, MD, Gary Null, PhD, and Debora Rasio, MD. "Death By Medicine," *Nexus New Times*, 11, no. 5. Refer to website: www.nutritioninstituteofamerica.org

11. "Strong warning on antidepressants urged," *The Seattle Times*, September 15, 2004.

what is occurring within the energy field of the individual experiencing the symptoms.

I have barely touched upon the many and varied treatment options available, but I am merely attempting to draw attention to the numerous choices available and the decisions needed when ill health occurs. I hear countless stories about the drawn-out process of getting an accurate diagnosis and then the numerous decisions needed for treatment options. For the average person who has little or no knowledge of physiology, anatomy, and other health-related matters, it has to be somewhat like trying to navigate his or her way through a complex and challenging maze.

By the way, it should be noted that current language usage refers to non-allopathic modalities as being "complementary," "alternative," or "integrative," which they may well be when used in conjunction with or instead of allopathic medicine—assuming that we use allopathic medicine as the baseline for healing! The truth is that many holistic modalities have been in use in different societies worldwide for longer than allopathic medicine has been practiced. It seems that these holistic modalities should be more accurately referred to as natural or traditional therapies.

In the previous chapter I stated that both healing and illness occur from the outside of the energy field and work inward until it manifests in the physical body. The interconnection between the physical body and the energy field is the reason for this. I will now explain in simplistic terms how this occurs. I have included common experiences and situations to highlight my position.

Energy Needs and Interactions

We rely on our energy levels for vitality and stamina every day. Sometimes energy levels can be high and we have excess; other times they become depleted and consequently we feel tired and lethargic. The energy source that sustains us is our energy field, which ultimately is our connection to the larger universal energy domain. It literally provides whatever energy is needed each day.

Whatever is experienced in life is initially felt in the energy field. An example of this occurs when you interact with someone for the first time. Instinctually you receive a sense of his or her character. Is this person trustworthy, likeable, and interesting? Or do you immediately become wary of this person's intentions? Your energy field connects with theirs and from that you are able to glean information about them. All this happens rapidly and intuitively, but, nevertheless, within the space of a few seconds you may often have a fairly reliable picture of the person's character.

Often a similar feeling occurs when you visit specific places. You may even experience a reaction of extreme comfort or discomfort. The vibes "out there" immediately register in your energy field and subtly, though not necessarily consciously, you sense what is occurring. Have you ever been some place and suddenly felt a shift in energies? In some instances it is highly likely that you are visiting a place that once was home to people of other cultures. Off the coast of Western Australia, there is an island that is a popular tourist destination. Rottnest Island was also once home to an indigenous aboriginal population. Even nowadays there are parts of Rottnest Island where the energies change dramatically, reflecting areas where conflict occurred between the indigenous aboriginal people and white settlers.

Another energy awareness situation occurs when you feel a strong instant connection with someone you have just met. Here, I am not only referring to that exciting sexual spark that ignites when you meet someone really special. The person you may feel an instant genuine liking for is most likely on the same wavelength as you are and may be of any culture, age, race, religion, or either sex. Remember that energy vibrates at varying frequencies. This means your energy field holds a certain vibration, and, when it connects with someone of a similar frequency, there is the likelihood of an almost instantaneous recognition. Again, the knowing and acceptance occurs outside your physical body. It immediately registers in the energy field. As your energy field nears that of other people or places, it reacts and responds to what it senses. Your energy field is continually active, providing feedback and giving off information, as well as connecting with other energy masses. It is never static.

Whatever emotions, thoughts, beliefs, and attitudes you hold about life are contained within your energy field, with the layers acting and reacting according to memories stored within while simultaneously responding to present stimuli. Other people easily sense everything stored within your energy field. Regarding the emotion of anger, the Dalai Lama is reported as saying "other people can sense it. It is almost as if they can feel steam coming out of the person's body."[12] It is the same with any other emotion. You intuitively and rapidly assess the emotion of people you interact with and then respond accordingly.

The energy field operates both as a transmitter and receiver. People, issues, and experiences that resonate with the energy frequencies you transmit are attracted to your energies. This means that in the course of a day the average person transmits and receives a mix of both positive and negative energies.

How Energy Impacts

When you experience considerable negativity in your life, this impacts harmfully on your energy levels. Consequently, your daily energy supplies may be rapidly depleted. Negativity arises from emotions, thoughts, and issues that create despondency, fear, or anger. In some instances, negative experiences are the result of a karmic cycle. Over a period of time of continual energy depletion, ill health is likely to occur. Energetically, you will always attract what you give out. So should you have emotions, such as anger, resentment, hatred, and judgment, the energy around these emotions returns to your energy field and affects its balance and functioning.

The human body is an incredibly complex machine and has the storage capacity of many computers. Everything you ever think, say, or do registers within your memory bank. Over time many negative experiences hold considerable weight as they impact and distort the energy

12.   Dalai Lama and Howard C. Cutler, MD. *The Art of Happiness*, Riverhead Books, 1998.

field. The finely spaced grid-like structure that makes up the energy field changes shape according to what is experienced. The fine silken threads weaken and then break in many places, gradually compressing into a mass, thereby making it difficult or even impossible for the microscopic golden balls of energy to move about. This is otherwise known as an energy blockage.

The energy of any experience takes up space within the layers of the energy field. Gradually, as beliefs and negative thinking continue throughout life, there is a buildup of this negative mind matter and they then permeate through the layers. This continues until they are eventually lodged in the physical body. From that, some form of bodily discomfort, distress, or illness manifests. Negative energy is destructive and toxic in so many ways. It not only hurts those at whom you may direct it, but it eventually returns home to bring some degree of pain.

Another form of energy depletion occurs when time is spent with people who function with a low daily energy supply. It is these people that are often described as "draining your energies." How often have you had the experience of being with someone who leaves you feeling depleted? After spending time with someone like this, it is inevitable that you will question where your vitality has gone. The practice of ensuring energy protection is covered in section 3.

There are other experiences and substances that, over time, have a detrimental impact upon the energy field. Every day you are exposed to a variety of substances that are considered acceptable and a normal part of life. Many of these substances are not beneficial to the energy field. They include alcohol, tobacco, drugs, caffeine, and chemicals that are inhaled and ingested, including environmental pollutants. Electromagnetic frequencies and extremely low frequency waves also have an impact upon the energy field.

On the other hand, positive thoughts, actions, and feelings generate further positive energy. The more you work with positive feelings and attitudes, the less time there is to expend on negativity. Consequently, life becomes less of a negative experience. Positive feelings and attitudes create a strong and bright energy field. This is because positive thoughts of love, compassion, peace, joy, harmony, and so on are beneficial to the energy field. Positive experiences and positive living strengthen, not deplete, the energy field. These reinforce the fine silky threads that are intricately woven within the web of the energy field, thereby enabling the minute golden balls of energy to do their work.

Role of the Chakra System

The chakra system is an integral aspect of the energy field and has a specific and critical purpose. Chakras are energy centers that store information drawn from life experiences and are located along the midline of the body, in both front and back. Much of the available literature focuses on the seven core chakras, which are divided into two distinct areas. The lower three chakras are about the physical or external world, and the upper three are about the inner or spiritual world. They are connected via the fourth chakra, or heart center, which is about humanitarian, unconditional love. In order to fully integrate the external and internal worlds, the heart center must be opened. This is a process that occurs as spiritual awareness takes place within the individual.

The function of chakras is to provide energy to the physical body and energy field, to develop awareness of the true self, and to act as a conduit for energy as it travels between the different layers within the energy field. The chakras form a holistic system, and, when blockages occur within them, they impact health and well-being. Daily stresses, emotional issues, and mental and spiritual confusion create blockages within chakras. Blockages may occur partially or completely in some or all chakras and are the result of how you feel about yourself and other people. When healing takes place, chakra blockages are released and the energy field is realigned and balanced. Generally, any form of bodywork is conducive to releasing energy blockages.

As you become more aware of your chakras and energy field, you will find an increase in conscious awareness as each chakra is fully opened (activated). This leads to awareness of your internal world, your inner spiritual being, and this in turn leads to sensitivity to other people.

While there has been great emphasis and focus on the seven chakras, it should be noted that there are countless energy centers, or vortices, in your body. As spiritual evolvement occurs, more and more of these chakras are activated, and they assist in fully integrating the spiritual level into all aspects of daily life. This information goes beyond what is generally taught and accepted. My teachers from other dimensions have shown me that the human body is capable of holding unlimited, activated chakras in all parts of the body.

Healing from the Outside

In terms of healing work, many traditional and natural healing practitioners understand the principle of working from the outside (energy field) in order to heal the inner (physical). Clearing and balancing the energy field means the way is then paved for the physical body to heal. Natural healing practitioners who are able to clear chakras and release energy blockages can assist in healing your energy field. However, eventually the preferred option is to be able to do this for yourself with a minimum of time and effort. Even better, the ultimate aim should be to have all chakras clear of blockages, balanced, and in alignment along with a strong healthy energy field.

Ultimately, it is always the body that heals itself. The body only needs the right conditions for this to occur. All practitioners of healing, irrespective of their training, merely assist the body's self-healing process. This fact seems largely forgotten in Western society due to the heavy reliance on skilled specialists for healing purposes. Regardless of whatever route is followed when ill health occurs, real healing only ever occurs over time when the individual focuses positive intent on healing.

There is a great deal that can be done consciously to create perfect health and harmony within your body. What I will be advocating in later chapters is achievable for anyone. The information shared is not new. It is really a matter of reconnecting with some very basic skills and practices. By applying them daily and consistently, your quality of life and health will be greatly enhanced.

Creating Awareness and Intention

The following exercise asks that you focus on what has happened in your life. The aim is to create awareness and understanding, in order to eventually create new pathways of thought and emotion.

Awareness Processing

This exercise is best done in a seated position. Ensure you are sitting comfortably with both feet on the floor.

Focus energy on your breath—inhale and exhale slowly and gently. Allow your mind to empty of chatter. Continue relaxed breathing. Now, bring your attention to some aspect of your life you would like to change or improve. Leave your mind out of this; instead allow the issue or situation to arise within your consciousness. Allow it to sit there and then observe it objectively, as if you are an outsider. Look at the issue or situation closely. Ask, "What have I done to create or contribute to this?" Then wait, keep your mind clear of conscious thought, and you will find the answer will come from deep within you. Trust what comes to you, even if it seems bizarre or unexpected.

Follow this process for any issue or situation that you seek to change. I recommend keeping a journal of issues and the resultant insights. In time a clear picture will emerge of behaviors, responses, beliefs, and perceptions. This exercise will assist you to have awareness around your role in the creation of issues and situations. It does not provide you with the solution—it merely highlights how you have contributed to its creation. This is important, as it will provide a critical tool for implementing change.

CHAPTER SIX
Body as Barometer

"Recognize what is in your sight,
and that which is hidden from you
will become plain to you."
—The Nag Hammadi Library—

According to metaphysical teachings, there is an underlying spiritual reason and explanation for whatever occurs within the body. The work of metaphysical proponents has helped a large number of people come to greater understanding around the underlying emotional and mental issues that underpin the pain they're experiencing, as well as assisting them to make meaningful changes in their lives in order to heal.[13]

Every emotion and thought has an effect on the body. Even fleeting and unconscious thoughts can result in powerful outcomes. The phrase, "I'm sick of this. I need a holiday," used intermittently by a friend whenever work stresses were overwhelming resulted, time and again, in her succumbing to various ailments necessitating absenteeism from the workplace. The thought created both the sickness and the mini-vacation from work. Another woman shared her story. Physically in sound health, she nevertheless felt intense emotional responses to situations. She regularly used the phrase, "I'm heartbroken," whenever she heard of someone's misfortune. In time, a heart murmur was detected in her otherwise healthy body. These examples illustrate the body's responses to the messages that are sent to it via thoughts and emotions.

Public opinion, too, strongly shapes belief systems and health stories. How often do you hear someone saying, "Everyone in my family, or at work, has been ill with the flu. I'm bound to be next"? Invariably that is what happens. The media reports on the latest influenza virus about to impact the population, and people then engage in speculation on the likelihood of succumbing to it. Ingrained within societal beliefs is the inevitability of illness occurring, especially when a belief is held at the subconscious level that illness will strike. Again, the particular thoughts and emotions held by the individual creates the very conditions that are feared.

Nothing ever happens by chance. When you learn to observe closely and begin to see how seemingly insignificant things interconnect and actually weave a larger picture, you are well on the way to actually understanding how to heal your body.

---

13.   Louise Hay. *You Can Heal Your Life*, Hay House Inc., 1984. Annette Noontil. *The Body is the Barometer of the Soul*, McPherson's Printing Group, 1998.

The human body is truly a barometer of all emotions, thoughts, and beliefs. If you allow yourself a few moments to reflect, you will probably be able to identify situations where emotions and beliefs have created a particular response within your body. In some instances it may even seem as if the same story keeps repeating itself. This is because there is a message in the recurring incidents. They will continue repeating themselves in a similar form until you finally get the message and remedy the situation, whether it relates to lifestyle, diet, beliefs, or behavioral patterns.

Overall health of the physical body, emotions, and state of mind are familiar topics for the average person, especially as media advertising and reporting continually focus on aspects of these. There is another important facet to self-healing, which so far I've not dwelled upon but have referred to fleetingly. This is the spiritual expression of the self. Healing the physical, mental, and emotional levels is, without doubt, a Herculean task at the best of times. However, without healing taking place on a deeper spiritual level, any other healing will only have minimal and short-term benefits.

Everyone has an inner essence, soul, or spirit. It is this inner essence that attracts life situations and experiences for your highest good. We may not consciously realize that we invite the lessons needed to assist our spiritual growth. However, once this realization sets in, there is every incentive to learn life's lessons easily and rapidly. With ongoing awareness and practice, the learning becomes less painful and requires reduced effort. The intensity of emotion and pain reduces as understanding surfaces and healing takes place. Learning from life experiences is akin to undertaking a journey to a new destination. The unknown road lies ahead prior to setting out on the journey. You can choose a road that is bumpy and filled with hazardous and nerve-wracking detours, resulting in discomfort and stress along the route. Or you can select the road that is relatively flat and straight. Doubtless, there are times when the detours look interesting and may be well worth exploring. That is ultimately a matter of choice.

We incarnate into each lifetime with the express purpose of growing more spiritually aware and to becoming aligned with a greater consciousness. During infancy we retain a memory of this but the process of inhabiting a dense physical body eventually limits our memory. As we grow into young children, we assimilate into the culture and ways of the earth plane. In some ways it could be said that a veil is placed over our earlier consciousness and with this placement we forget the reasons for choosing to experience another lifetime in the human form.

The process of self-healing, if it is to be successful, must in some way integrate the true spiritual self with the physical reality and the perception of self. This necessitates detachment from the ego, which is more a mind perception of who one is. By this I mean it is easy to label yourself as a successful architect or pharmacist, or whatever else you chose to identify with, and to view the world purely from that perspective. These labels are a veneer or veil covering the core of your inner essence or soul. Defining who you are through the ego involves attachment to a material world where success is measurable and where competition and separatism predominate.

Accessing the inner essence involves peeling back the layers of the veil that were placed, consciously and subconsciously, within the psyche. The longer those layers have been submerged, the more challenging it becomes to remove them. The reason for this is that as physical reality predominates, there is less focus on developing and maintaining regular and meaningful spiritual practice. Generally, within Western society, the focus of daily attention, time, and energy is devoted to tangible and real situations. A consensus belief assumes that reality is measurable, quantifiable, and concrete.

Often a major paradigm shift is necessary before an individual begins to really question the meaning of life. This commonly occurs when a major illness or disaster strikes. It may also arise when the person continually feels dissatisfaction with aspects of life, realizing that old and familiar habits no longer feel comfortable or acceptable. An element of inner restlessness begins to ferment, which generally impacts all areas of a previously stable and comfortable existence. This is a sign from the inner essence, an indication that harbingers significant change.

When this occurs, it is most likely an uncomfortable and often distressing experience, as the individual questions and reacts in unpredictable and emotional ways to situations that in the past have been calmly accepted. Intense emotional reactions and inner pain are indicators that the veils of illusion are beginning to lift. Their removal can be likened to peeling away layers of dead skin. Snakes readily shed their skin; they innately know when it is time to do so. Human beings, on the other hand, love their attachments, and, when the inner essence, or soul, decides to shed an old skin that has outlived its usefulness, the ego resists. So the internal conflict begins and continues for as long as is necessary in order for the soul to be truly felt, heard, and responded to.

This generally results in a great number of life changes for the individual—some of those physical, many emotional and mental. The most important change, though, is the exploration of the inner world, an inner world that has far more depth, dimension, and reality to it than the outer physical reality. When this begins, there is an opportunity for real and lasting healing to occur.

Do not be under the illusion that when such inner conflict occurs the inner spirit always emerges victorious. Life continuously offers choice in all things. For some people, dealing with inner pain or exploring their inner essence is too uncomfortable. When this is the case, there are socially acceptable means readily available to dull the senses and emotions. The most common of these are listed below. The need for each is likely to become addictive, either physically or psychologically, when used regularly as a means of escaping the dreariness and pain of life.

- Regular alcohol consumption offers a means of anaesthetizing pain when life issues become too stark and confronting.

- Prescription medications, especially antidepressants and other mood and behavior modifiers, are commonly used and widely accepted.

- Individuals often claim cigarette smoking provides a means of coping with stress.

- Recreational drugs offer the user an opportunity to experience an altered mind state, thereby creating a temporary and bearable reality.

- Caffeine consumption provides a temporary lift in energy, which psychologically enhances perceptions of reality.

There is a damaging impact upon the energy field from the regular use and consumption of these substances. For many people, situations arise that result in pain. This pain is often not dealt with. It may be suppressed or denied by the individual, who may lack appropriate coping skills. Instead, the emotional or mental pain remains within the energy field, resulting in the formation of energy blockages. At a deeper level the pain persists, and so the soul quietly reminds the individual of the discomfort that is felt due to the energy blockage. The individual, for whatever reason, chooses instead one or more of the above-mentioned substances to ease the discomfort. Often the pain or discomfort presents itself as a vague uneasiness and dissatisfaction with life, and the resultant quick fix is to mask the pain with a substance that is readily available.

The actual energy grid that comprises the structure of the energy field is already experiencing distress due to the blockage from the stored emotional or mental pain. The fine silken threads are no longer finely and evenly spaced, and the golden balls of energy are unable to move as they are designed to do. Instead the silken threads are clumped together, impeding the free flow of energy. The energy flow has had to adjust to and accommodate this blockage, so already there is some degree of damage suffered within the energy field.

When toxins are inhaled and ingested as a means of obviating pain, further damage occurs to the energy grid. All the substances listed above are lethal to the energy grid. The sensitive silken threads wither when exposed to toxins. They lose their vitality, strength, and flexibility and become misshapen and dramatically weakened. This process is gradual and compounds the problems created by the existing blockage due to previously stored pain. Inevitably a lifetime of unhealed pain combined with regular toxin exposure will result in an energy grid that is unable to function healthily and strongly. Ill health is inevitable.

Whenever pain is experienced on the emotional, mental, or spiritual levels, there is a subtle shift in the normal and healthy functioning of the energy grid, resulting in a lack of balance. If the suffering is not healed, in time symptoms manifest, usually as mild aches or some degree of discomfort within the physical body. This is the body's way of signaling that there is something amiss. It is a gentle reminder, sent via your body, that it is time to take healing action because some aspect of your life is discordant. Most people are readily able to identify the issues causing the discomfort. In many instances the core issues are mental or emotional in nature and relate to relationship or work issues. They may also be in some way connected to their deeper search for meaning.

Often it is easy to identify an issue as being either emotional or mental in origin, when, on an even deeper level, it actually is an expression of the soul. The emergence of the inner essence, or soul, manifests in many ways. Soul has a voice and clamors to be heard. It will not desist, regardless of your response to its message. Experiencing inner turmoil and physical pain is a sign from your soul that something in your life needs to be looked at and healed. Your soul loves to be in a permanent state of peace and harmony. It savors balance and bliss. It thrives on positive attitude and loving energies. The struggling and resistance ceases and from there, feelings of well-being permeate the energy field.

Acknowledging the soul and allowing its light to shine outwardly is an integral aspect of self-healing. The body is truly the barometer of the inner essence or soul. Whenever your soul is in pain, it reflects outwardly and ultimately manifests in a tangible form, which can then be recognized and corrected. The importance of recognizing and acknowledging the soul is critically essential to the self-healing steps I will be outlining in the following chapters.

Intuitive Allowing

This visualization exercise is intended to bring to your awareness the reasons or causes of any previous illness or condition you may have experienced. It does not involve undertaking a healing process. Rather this is intended to create awareness and understanding. Later exercises will include healing visualizations, along with practical strategies.

1. *Find a quiet space; sit comfortably with feet placed firmly on the ground and arms resting lightly in your lap. Close your eyes and begin breathing quietly, deeply, and slowly. Focus attention on your breath until you clear the chatter in your mind.*

2. *Once you are in a calm and quiet space, allow your focus on breathing to become less prominent, though continue having awareness of the movement of the breath within your body.*

3. *Slowly bring to your consciousness an illness or condition that has affected you at some time in your life. As you bring the memory to your consciousness, observe it without bringing in any of the emotions. This places you in a position of being the outsider who observes events, issues, and emotions without having any involvement.*

4. *Observe the onset of the illness or condition. What were your feelings at the time? What was happening in your life?*

5. *Then bring your consciousness back further—six months, twelve months, and even earlier. Consciously locate whatever created the illness or condition. Was there a significant event that triggered a response?*

6. *Look for a cause and effect situation. Observe your emotions and reactions. Can you understand the reason for these? Where do your emotions and reactions originate?*

7. *Continue consciously exploring whatever is revealed to you while in this relaxed state and without emotion. Ask questions and then wait for the answers to be revealed. They may be revealed as a vivid scene or possibly as something that you immediately know.*

8. *A picture will emerge from the questioning that will provide clues regarding the origin of whatever illness or condition you seek to understand. From this you will begin to see the link between your mental and emotional states and the resultant illness or condition that occurred.*

This exercise can also be used to explore life situations that have caused you pain. You may find that inadvertently making a certain statement repeatedly has resulted in illness. Or you may discover that suppressed emotions of anger have resulted in difficulties in relationships. The causes and effects are countless. However, gaining awareness and understanding of the link is vital to releasing and healing the pain.

HEALING
PRINCIPLES

CHAPTER SEVEN
Creating Meaningful Change

*"You are never given a wish without also
being given the power to make it true."*
—*Richard Bach*—

The self-healing principles and practices I advocate will be explored in greater depth in this section of the book. As you will discover, there is nothing radically new in what is shared. However, the emphasis and focus, in many instances, will be slightly different than what is generally expounded. It is my intention to create another way of viewing the world. In other words, I hope to create new and exciting perceptions and assist in the creation of a paradigm shift. My understanding, through my own healing experiences and working with clients, is that it is important to:

- become completely aware and mindful of all that you do.
- be clear about your intentions.
- see and understand the signs or messages in all that happens.

Having this degree of mindfulness and awareness in everyday life will greatly assist in creating a shift in perception, thus producing a paradigm shift. This is not to suggest that there is a need to become paranoid or self-obsessed about every particular detail or incident—far from it. Rather, it is hoped that the information shared here encourages you to question more deeply aspects of life you are not satisfied with and seek to change. I hope to inspire you to make meaningful changes to improve the quality of your life. Maybe the information and suggestions for creating wellness will help you deal with life differently and in a more positive and empowering manner.

Quite a number of years ago I read an inspiring book, the title of which has long since been forgotten, but part of its message is still vividly clear. This book explored in depth three distinct personality categories. My summation here is concise but serves to explain what I'm endeavoring to share.

The first personality type was depicted as a shark. The shark is a predator, has a predisposition to be aggressive, and will push relentlessly to achieve desired goals. When there are obstructions, the shark will be more determined than ever to succeed. However, when confronting obstacles, the characteristic behavior of the shark is to continue doing more of the same but even harder. If something doesn't work initially, the only real option is to continue doing more of the same but with greater exertion.

The second personality category was another fish type, for convenience let's call it a mackerel. A mackerel is the exact opposite of the shark. It is timid, hesitant, and when confronted by aggression and obstacles, it will cede territory. The mackerel has no real backbone, is a "yes" personality, has no real opinion on current trends, and is often on the receiving end of the shark's intimidating and bullying behavior.

The dolphin represented the third personality category. The dolphin is neither shark nor mackerel but has the characteristics of both. It knows when to be assertive and strong, when to attack, and also when to retreat. This personality type uses his or her intelligence to assess situations and is then in the ideal position to react accordingly. Dolphins respond after thinking things through rather than reacting emotionally or instinctively. The dolphin personality assesses all possibilities, will be hard-nosed when necessary, or will acquiesce when it is strategically advantageous. When something is not working as anticipated, the dolphin personality reassesses the situation and instead of continuing even more determinedly in the same manner will look to other possible, easier, solutions. The dolphin personality is a lateral and creative thinker, in tune with emotions but not controlled by them.

In all likelihood you can identify with these three personality types. There may be times when you wear the shark's garb and unleash whatever aggression and determination is necessary to achieve your goals. Such responses are often instinctual or learned; you truly believe or know this is the only way to achieve desired outcomes. Other times, when confronted by another even more determined shark personality, it is prudent to withdraw. Again, such a response is most likely instinctual. In such situations you are likely to exhibit the timid behavior of the mackerel.

Ideally, you would aspire to have the wisdom, strength, and tenacity of the dolphin. It would be easy to believe that the dolphin personality matches your responses to life situations at all times, though truthfully that is highly unlikely. It would be easy to deny vehemently that shark or mackerel behaviors or attitudes in any way influence your life choices. In reality, all individuals exhibit the behaviors and responses instinctual to all three personality categories. Similarly, our responses to issues, people, and situations are based on more than only the immediate circumstances confronting us.

My suggestion is that you adopt the dolphin personality characteristics as you read and begin to implement the strategies and changes suggested in the following chapters. Instead of reacting as a shark or mackerel, apply the dolphin's strategic thinking and planning skills. As you commence this process, you may wish to adopt the following steps.

1. Assess your current lifestyle habits without making any judgments.

2. Where you find dissatisfaction and would like to make improvements, evaluate where and how this can be achieved with a minimum of discomfort or pain in order to achieve the maximum benefit.

3. Allow time to adjust to any implemented changes before progressing to the next step. This way you will be in a position to smoothly integrate new concepts and ways of perceiving, modify behaviors, and so on.

4. You are in charge of the process, and as the benefits begin to become evident, you will feel empowered to continue.

This is your journey to create wellness, which involves a steady process of change and growth. You are at the helm and can choose where and how to map your course. With each success, no matter how small or large, you will find the inner encouragement to proceed further. To begin manifesting change positively, it is important to have awareness of how your energy and attention are focused culturally. By having clarity and awareness around this, you are in a position to create a reality that is more aligned with your real—and not perceived—desires and goals.

External Influences

Life in Western society tends to be structured in such a way that a great deal of individual time and effort is expended on what I refer to as "externals." The need to earn income to pay the rent or mortgage as well as the bills that arrive with unremitting regularity is what keeps most people motivated. It often seems like being on a never-ending treadmill. The daily routine is get up, go to work, shop, and run errands after work. After that, if there is spare time or inclination, there is the possibility for leisure activities in the evening before going to bed. Most people in Western societies believe and accept that this is how life is meant to be lived. Of course, this description is hugely oversimplified, but I'm sure the meaning is clear. Daily demands are increasingly time-consuming, thereby limiting opportunity for exploring other options. Basically, these external demands dominate, determine, and shape general lifestyle choices.

Western culture focuses enormous attention on individual physical appearance and attributes as well as the general image portrayed. Value and importance are placed on external beauty and success. Learning to judge others and ourselves by outward appearances commences from an early age. If ever you were to seriously question the role that advertising, whether blatant or subtle, plays on your self-perception, I'm sure you would be greatly shocked by its level of influence.

For example, constant advertising on the efficacy of different diets bombards the consumer via various media outlets. The underlying message is twofold. First, the purpose of advertising is to convince the consumer of the value of a product. Advertising aims to sell. That is the first and only reason advertising exists! Second, by implication the general public is told there is something wrong with their shape and weight. A perusal of any popular magazine clearly demonstrates this point.

Advertising language and messages are so subtle, yet powerful, that the individual is encouraged to diet because it is promoted as helpful to overall health. There is no denying that a healthy, nutritious diet, along with lifestyle changes, will result in weight and body shape changes. But that is not the reason advertising promotes the many different diets now being promulgated by the mass media. The media gives continual reminders on the importance of focusing on the externals. The emphasis is that your body shape and size, irrespective of how you actually feel and look, are in need of modification, and once this is achieved, instant health and happiness are attained. If only it were that easy!

The same applies to another habit constantly encouraged within our society: amassing the latest offerings in material goods. Societal conditioning and beliefs hold that acquiring the latest and fastest technological products will enhance the quality of life. Emphasis is placed on continually updating and upgrading homes, cars, and all the paraphernalia deemed necessary for existence. This pursuit of consumerism is greater now than at any other time in history. Culturally it has become acceptable to value external appearances and material consumerism as the *modus operandi*.

Change and Consequences

Technology has certainly changed life dramatically in the last fifty years or so with earlier generations living in a time of less complexity. Many of the homespun principles and values taught by earlier generations have as much relevance today as they did then. The focus in previous generations was still on survival—earning sufficient income and being able to creatively ensure that survival was reasonably comfortable. The major difference between then and now is that we are rapidly becoming totally reliant on external sources for survival. Traditional wisdom and many basic living skills are being lost as public dependence on multinational corporations increasingly provides the individual with his or her daily needs.

Reliance on external factors applies to both consumer habits and personal lives. There is a tendency to look to others for guidance and direction, generally trusting their perception of how the world is rather than relying on your inner knowing. It is common to blame others when life deals a poor hand. Looking to other people, often family, institutions, or public figures, to sort out problems is a commonly accepted practice. On yet another level, even God is perceived as an external being, someone who for unknown reasons may have caused pain or great disasters.

Somehow, in embracing a consumer-oriented and technologically expansive way of life, it has become all too easy for individuals to be disassociated and separated from their inner knowing, wisdom, and strength. It has become acceptable to abrogate responsibility for all that happens as life becomes focused on externals. This is not how earlier generations understood the world. Theirs was predicated on inner wisdom and knowing. They came to know themselves intimately and realized that knowing came from within, that survival was an inner process, and that the Creator was within everything on this planet, including them.

This is not to suggest that a reversion to former times and conditions is preferred. There is so much information available nowadays that can assist us to move from living a totally external focused life to creating a life of balance, one where inner wisdom guides our actions, beliefs, and choices.

Historically, we are in a time of increasing conscious awareness. This is an opportunity to come to know a great deal more about ourselves and universal truths. We can also choose to remain living in a world that is focused mainly on the externals and refrain from looking more deeply into our current reality. However, the fact that you are reading these words suggests you are ready to embrace change in some aspect of your life.

Change Process

Change is inevitable. Most people comment on the rapid rate of change occurring in their lives. In some instances change results from individual initiative. In most cases, however, change is forced on the individual. Change occurs for physical, mental, emotional, and spiritual reasons. It is not necessary to actually define the reason nor is in-depth analysis actually needed. However, having some understanding of the issues and process will assist greatly. Whenever change occurs in your life, on any level, there are steps you can take to facilitate the process:

1. Accept that change will occur at different times throughout life. Resisting change requires a lot of mental and emotional energy. Change will occur, irrespective of your feelings. Resistance is futile and only results in added stress.

2. Observe and assess change as it occurs. Take note of what is actually happening. How can you ease the changes comfortably into your life? What are the consequences? How can the impact be minimized? What are the best ways of working with the process?

3. Apply the skills and strategies of the dolphin personality. Be creative, use your intuition, and think laterally when problems arise during the change process. Look for obvious solutions that will work. Doing the same thing repeatedly with more intensity (common behavior of the shark personality) does not work in times of change.

4. Find the positive aspects in whatever change is occurring and focus on them. Then look beyond each positive and see what other advantages can be created from the change.

5. Work with the change process, rather than against it. Take it one step at a time and focus your energy and intent on that particular step. Doing this means that the whole process does not feel as arduous or stressful.

6. Finally, learn to embrace change. Welcome it into your life. Change fosters growth and increases awareness. It provides learning opportunities and can enhance confidence.

In the following chapters I will be focusing on traditional wisdom for well-being as it applies in the modern world. There will be a meshing and interweaving of the physical with the spiritual. Emphasis will be placed on intuitive knowing and listening to the inner voice in order to determine what is the best possible way of healing and living life positively. By following the practical healing exercises and suggestions, you will come to a greater understanding of how your current life has been created. If you desire to make changes, you will learn how this can be manifested.

As I wrote earlier, all I share is straightforward. We are now living in a time when the resources, knowledge, and ability to make meaningful and lasting change in all areas of life are readily accessible and available. We can collectively change the course of history, from one of confrontation and enmity to one of global peace and harmony.

Years ago I read a most profound piece of wisdom that basically states, "If you want to change the world, change yourself." You have nothing to lose but everything to gain when you begin to put into effect some of the basic principles I've found to be extremely powerful in creating change for empowerment and well-being.

Strategy for Creating Meaningful Change

As you read the following chapters you may wish to initiate some changes, significant or otherwise, in your life. Before reading any further I suggest that you quietly reflect on your current life situation. Take a few moments to still your mind and focus on any desired change. Focus on where you are now and then imagine how you will be once the intended change has been implemented. Now, it is time to begin planning. I suggest using pen and paper or computer to jot down your strategy for creating the change you desire. This process can be applied to practically all areas of change you choose to implement.

1. Clearly identify the area of change intended. If you are generally dissatisfied with your life, identify exactly the aspects you wish to change. For example, you may intend to create better social and interpersonal skills, or you may anticipate strengthening a particular friendship or relationship. Be clear and concise about your intended change, as this provides the basis for creating the steps necessary for implementing the actual change.

2. Once you have clearly identified the change or goal, write it down. Now you have the opportunity to daydream and imagine! Allow your mind to explore the many possible ways your goal can be achieved. Write down all the possibilities imagined, irrespective of how inane or insane they may seem. If you feel stuck at this stage,

ask someone you trust for assistance. Often, another person can offer unexpected and plausible suggestions.

3. Assess the list of possible steps you have written down. Which ones feel right to implement? Are there any possible unintended consequences that could arise from any of those listed? This is the stage where you need to be analytical. Carefully scrutinize each possibility listed and determine which ones will work and then place them into a feasible working order.

4. Prioritize your possibilities. Is there any one step that must be implemented first? Can you see a sequence for working through the steps in order to create the change you are seeking? If so, write down the sequence. Then leave the list for a day or so.

5. After you have had time for reflection, read over what you have already created. This time lag will enable you to review what you have identified with greater objectivity and clarity. Reassess your list. Make any modifications you feel are necessary. Add, delete, and change until you are satisfied with your creation. This is the list of steps you will take to create the desired changes. This list should basically comprise things to do.

6. It may be necessary to break each of the steps into even smaller bite-sized pieces. There may be several smaller aspects that need to be dealt with within the larger step. Identify where this is the case and then list each of the smaller steps accordingly. You are gradually creating a plan of action. By having all the necessary steps clearly identified, you will save yourself a lot of guesswork and will be able to meaningfully structure the change process for your needs.

7. Write a plan of action, including all the steps to be implemented. Also include a time frame so that you have a clear and workable structure.

8. Implement the action plan. Refer back to your plan regularly. Be clear about achieving each of the steps you have set for yourself. Focus on one step at a time. That way you will not be easily

discouraged. As you progress, you may find that changes are necessary to the action plan; make those changes as needed.

9. You may also choose to journal the change process or to record your experiences in some way. This is an affirming and confidence-building exercise.

10. Finally, reward yourself for your persistence and achievement. Creating the change you intended could probably be regarded as sufficient reward. However I suggest you actually reward yourself with something that gives you enjoyment. You deserve a reward for your determination and success.

CHAPTER EIGHT
Food for Healing

*"Those who do not find some time for
health must sacrifice
a lot of time one day for illness."*
—Sebastian Kniepp—

Hippocrates, founder of modern medicine, is quoted as saying, "Everyone has a doctor in him or her; we just have to help it in its work. The natural healing force within each one of us is the greatest force in getting well. Our food should be our medicine. Our medicine should be our food. But to eat when you are sick is to feed your sickness."[14] I believe most people have either lost sight of this concept or are totally unaware of its relevance to daily life. This is largely because there is so much conflicting advertising and hype about food, diet, and healthy eating choices.

It is important to examine the actual meaning of this statement. Food provides sustenance and nourishment for the physical body. It produces physical energy and ensures optimal performance on a daily basis, in addition to providing essential nutrients to cells for healthy functioning. Earlier I referred to the energy field and its critical role in ensuring that there is sufficient energy sustenance throughout the day. When there is depletion in the energy field, there is attendant loss in energy and well-being. In much the same way, the physical body requires food as its fuel source. Good quality food is critical to healthy functioning of the body. The information in this chapter and the next will explain the importance of ensuring that the foods you consume are healthy. Premium quality food is critical for the healing process and for maintaining health on the physical level.

Food as Medicine

Hippocrates asserted that food should be our medicine. Basically this means that whatever food is ingested should maintain your body in a healthy state. Ideally, the food you consume should always be of the highest quality in order to facilitate the functioning of a strong, lean, and lithe body.

There are some general eating patterns and perceptions held about food within our society. As a general rule, you only eat when you are hungry. If only that were the truth! If you are like the majority of people, you eat because you believe you are hungry. You have been conditioned to

---

14. www.quotationspage.com/quotes/Hippocrates.

believe a minimum of three meals a day is essential, and your body has become accustomed to that habit. Newborn babies demand food when they are hungry due to an internal mechanism that registers hunger. Over time this mechanism regulates into a reasonable routine. However, have you ever noticed that young children have a less defined feeding schedule? Their bodies still tell them when they're hungry, when they're not hungry, and what they're hungry for. Babies and young children naturally listen to the needs and demands of their body and will not hesitate to make those needs known.

Adults generally have lost this ability of discrimination. Instead, meals are eaten like clockwork. Desired foods are chosen regardless of the body's needs. This is because the average adult has become accustomed to certain food preferences and dietary lifestyles. From time to time I see this with clients whose eating habits have the potential to become a major contributor of their ultimate cause of death. Weight gain, heart attacks, arthritis, food allergies, and digestive disorders are some of the numerous conditions common to clients. In many instances, clients know that dietary changes would result in improved health but are reluctant to live without their favorite foods.

Food is a common social lubricator. There is no shortage of holidays and celebrations where food predominates. These provide a wonderful opportunity for socializing with family and friends. As well, the sharing of a meal offers a common ground for business and political gatherings. Social and cultural conditioning encourages you to focus your life around food. Eating large portions is also culturally accepted and encouraged. The advent of fast-food outlets and buffet-style eating has certainly supported this dietary change.

Consequently, it seems the practice of relying on being in a state of actual hunger before eating has either been discarded or lost. This means that eating only to appease hunger and being discriminating about what is necessary for your body's health and well-being are also becoming extinct practices. Please note that these are broad generalizations. There always have been people who view food from a perspective that is aligned with their body's preferences and needs. Sadly, however, such people are not the vast majority of the population.

A brief look at the average population supports my concerns. Statistics reported in the news media indicate that over 60 percent of the American population has a weight problem, with obesity on the increase. Solutions abound for getting rid of the excess weight, ranging from all types of diet regimes to surgical stapling procedures. It is time to seriously question whether the foods that are generally consumed act as medicines generating healthy bodies or whether they actually contribute to the range of conditions and illnesses currently being experienced by many people.

If the foods eaten contain all the essential nutrients needed by the body, then overall good health should be expected. It stands to reason. Therefore it is reasonable to seriously question whether the foods available for consumption contain the necessary beneficial nutrients. Many customary and preferred foods are highly processed and contain quite a cocktail of additives and chemicals, all included to add flavor, enhance shelf life, and appeal to the consumer. In general, taste buds have become highly receptive to foods with added sweeteners and taste enhancers.

It has become customary for the average person to eat a range of snack foods that have little or no nutritional value. A culture has been created that espouses fast foods, including snack eating, loaded with empty calories. It is not surprising that the results of such indiscriminate eating patterns are now becoming apparent. Increased weight is only one consequence. Other conditions or illnesses result from ingesting highly processed foods that are laden with sugar, fats, additives, preservatives, and shelf life and flavor intensifiers.

Food Production Changes

Crop growing and food production have changed dramatically in the last one hundred years. Small farm lots seem to be the exception rather than commonplace. Agriculture has become highly mechanized and is now big business. The use of chemical fertilizers, herbicides, and pesticides continues to increase as arable land is farmed on a larger scale than ever before. It would be naïve to believe that all traces of these chemicals are completely removed from foods grown and processed.

There are long-term and residual effects of chemicals such as chlordane, DDT (dichlorodiphenyltrichloroethane), and PCBs (polychlorinated biphenyls), which are still found in measurable quantities in plant and animal life worldwide. PCBs have been banned for use in the United States in all but completely enclosed areas since 1979, but they still persist in the environment and in animal fat. All that is needed for contamination to occur is for this to be passed on through the food chain. An example of this occurs when insects are eaten by small fish, which in turn are eaten by larger fish. PCBs accumulate and are stored in body fat.

Larger fish, such as some farmed salmon, have been found in recent years to contain unacceptable levels of PCBs, which are endocrine disrupters. They can cause cancer, infertility, and even sexual changes. In the 1970s, when studying human ecology, I read of their damaging impact on the reproductive systems of animals. It seems many toxins that have been used indiscriminately are still found within environmental ecosystems and continue to create health problems.

The rapid technological changes made to food production and processing in the last fifty or so years have resulted in considerable changes to the foods actually consumed. The average citizen no longer knows what is in the foods they purchase. Labeling may assist in making some informed choices, but it does not necessarily tell what the different additives will eventually do to the body. There are no guarantees that added stress is not placed upon the body due to the chemicals contained in the foods we consume. Most likely there will be a cumulative overloading of toxins, which will result in ill health manifesting in one form or another.

Technology has made speedy advances in ensuring fresh food is delivered to local supermarkets. Shelf life has been enhanced dramatically, especially for foods that fifty years ago only had a short shelf life. There is no doubt that this has added considerable variety to the daily diet, but it has not necessarily added to the quality of the foods eaten. Many processed or treated foods (whether through irradiation or any other technological means) may look appealing and even taste delicious, but is there any guarantee that the nutritional value is retained?

Do you recall the tantalizingly sweet and juicy taste of homegrown fruits or vegetables that are naturally grown? They have a taste and flavor that is not replicated with mass-produced and genetically modified crops. In addition, picking crops when they are vine-ripened ensures the presence of monosaccharides, which are essential for healthy cell functioning and repair. Crops harvested prior to ripening on the plant lack this ingredient.

Growing food crops has become a highly industrialized and technical business. Scientific research and analysis have contributed enormously to the growth and expansion of the agricultural industry. Nowadays the practice of genetically modifying seeds and plants is gaining momentum worldwide. This, I have read, is to improve seed and crop quality, durability, and production output, as well as resistance to common insect and weed infestations. Eating genetically modified foods, however, is not without some risks. Genetically modified foods have not been proven safe for human consumption.

There have been outraged expressions and demonstrations from communities worldwide at the introduction of genetically modified foods into their food supplies. My reading of the literature has revealed there are implications for the human body when genetically modified foods are eaten. Studies indicate evidence of damage to the immune system and vital organs. It must be remembered that for years the general public was told hormone replacement therapy (HRT) was safe. It was the main medication prescribed to assist women through menopause. However, after many years of research, discussion, and debate, the latest findings demonstrate clearly that there is a considerable health risk associated with taking this medication. The study into genetically modified foods is still in its infancy but already the signs exist that it would be advisable to be wary of rushing into compliant acceptance of this further adulteration of the food system. It could very well be another potential HRT!

Increased Consumer Awareness

As a consumer you have the right to know what is in the food you purchase. You have the right to know when foods are genetically modified.

You have the right to demand knowledge of the real and long-term implications of eating food that has been changed or genetically modified in any way.

A great deal of research is continually being undertaken to assess the safety and efficacy of drugs and foods available for human consumption. Much of this research is undertaken by the industries actually producing these chemicals and products. For obvious reasons, it is vitally important that industries adhere to stringent safety standards and high-quality production. However, there should be a requirement that demands compulsory independent testing of all such products by a minimum of two agencies to confirm or deny the findings of company-initiated testing. As mentioned previously, agriculture and food production is big business, and a great deal of money is invested in garnishing a profitable market share. With this in mind, there should be a high degree of accountability for any product that is marketed to the general public. Independent research, assessment, analysis, and reporting of findings would go a long way toward keeping the consumer informed about what is really included in foods and other consumer products and to what extent modifications will affect long-term health.

Chemicals in Foods

There are already excess chemicals in the land, waterways, and air resulting in toxins that need to be eliminated by the body. These toxins have accumulated at an ever-increasing rate since the beginning of the Industrial Era. Recently I heard that the average person is currently exposed to approximately sixteen thousand chemicals on a daily basis. Toxic overload, or chemical hypersensitivity, is increasingly affecting people in industrialized societies. Their lives are difficult enough as they endeavor to find an accurate diagnosis for their condition. In addition, their lives require adaptation to minimize the effects of these noxious toxins that are found practically everywhere—in food, buildings, and local environments.

Overall, the state of health experienced within the general public is far from excellent. The foods eaten in an average diet, instead of being our medicine as prescribed by Hippocrates, are more than likely to contribute considerably to increasing ill health.

According to Phillip Day, most common illnesses and conditions are basically metabolic diseases, meaning that they can be attributed to nutritional deficiencies in the body.[15] Metabolic diseases cannot be cured by medication. Rather, they require a preventative, the lacking nutrients, that must be put back into the body. Taking the preventative involves a life-long commitment, otherwise the illness or condition will recur once the nutrition is withdrawn.

Food that is denatured does not support the physical body in cellular repair and connectivity. All toxins, whether ingested or inhaled, have an impact on the energy grid. Chemicals weaken the structure and formation of healthy and vital energy pathways. The process of gradual deterioration becomes marked over a period of time and eventually affects the physical body on a cellular level. The energy grid itself loses its solid structural formation as the web weakens and withers. A way to imagine this is to observe a beautifully woven spider's web. Its intricacy of structure is stunning. However, should you accidentally brush against the spider's web, a part of it will disintegrate and its wholeness is damaged. It is the same with your energy grid when it is continually exposed to chemicals and synthetic substances. This exposure occurs through a process of ingestion, inhalation, or absorption of toxins through the skin.

Medicine as Food

The second part of Hippocrates' quote, "Let our medicine be our food," bears scrutiny. Here he is basically saying that when you are ill or feeling unwell, the best treatment is the food you consume. Can you imagine a donut and coffee offering the best medicinal treatment?

Hippocrates lived in a time when food was not mass-produced and processed in factories. In ancient times meat was hunted, fish was caught, and fruits, vegetables, seeds, and spices would all have been

---

15.   Phillip Day. *Health Wars*, Credence Publications, 2001.

grown within the local vicinity. When food was needed, it was then hunted or gathered and consumed while still fresh. Simple methods for storage and preserving would have been used. Food would not have been kept in storage for months at a time, nor would it have been transported across countries or oceans, as is now common practice.

Hippocrates' statement could be interpreted as an indication that food grown locally, naturally, and in fertile soils is highly nutritious and therefore beneficial to the body. He understood how the body works and knew that the natural vitamins, minerals, enzymes, and amino acids found in foods are essential to tissue repair and healing. Quality, nutritious food works by fueling the body, assists with the oxygenation process, and creates balance and harmony internally. The liver, kidneys, and digestive system do not become overloaded or congested when food is easily metabolized and digested, which is the case when one eats naturally grown and produced foods. This means there is reduced stress on the body, and the body is then able to heal itself.

One of the conditions I often see when working with clients is liver overload. The liver is the super processor and toxin filter of the body. This wonder organ processes everything that is ingested. Considering that it is not unusual for the average person to eat three to five servings of food a day, drink several cups of coffee, a soda or two, imbibe in alcohol, inhale nicotine, take some form of medication, as well as inhaling and ingesting a myriad of environmental chemicals, it is little wonder that the average liver becomes congested and tired.

An overworked, congested liver quickly lets the body know it is stressed. The obvious solution is to make some beneficial changes to diet. This rests and cleanses the liver and assists the body to heal.[16] In most instances, people are not aware of this message their body is sending out. More likely they will blame work, family, or a relationship situation for the fact that they're continually tired, suffer with digestive problems, have allergies, or are unable to cope. By making healthy changes to diet, the body begins healing and functions better, and the individual then begins to feel more like their normal self.

---

16.   Dr. Sandra Cabot. *The Liver Cleansing Diet*, Women's Health Advisory Service, 1996.

Another two common conditions I encounter in clients' bodies are a weakened immune system and a compromised neurological system. These are very much a result of twentieth and twenty-first century living. The chemicals we are exposed to daily create mayhem within the body. As explained earlier, the body is a highly sensitive energy system. Toxins affect it and create a whole host of conditions that are damaging to it. Both the immune and neurological systems are integral to good health. They are sensitive, susceptible, and responsive to outside influences. Naturally, the body will always do all it can to self-heal. However, the gradual and continuous accumulation of toxins ultimately results in overload, thereby creating an environment where resistance to illness is further diminished.

It is essential to good physical and energetic health to ensure that the foods we eat are of a high quality and beneficial to the body. How else can the body's organs and general functioning repair and regenerate? In the following chapter I will share how easy it is to make changes to diet and a diet-related lifestyle to ensure that the body's exposure to toxins is reduced.

CHAPTER NINE

Natural
is Best

*"Facts do not cease to exist
because they are ignored."*
—Aldous Huxley—

My teachers from other dimensions have been responsible for sharing more than the principles of energy and healing. They have also guided and tutored me about the importance of honoring the physical body. One of the statements that has been repeated many times is "Natural is best." This statement actually refers to more than just food, but in this chapter I will share my understanding of how it relates mainly to diet and some aspects of personal care.

A broad overview was provided in the previous chapter of general trends in food production and consumption habits. An overview is all it is, which means it has limitations. A great deal more could have been included, but as the focus of this book is multifaceted, the generalities shared will hopefully inspire you to investigate further. It is my intention to create awareness and to stimulate further questioning about what actually happens in the food industry and the possible consequences for your long-term health based on current trends.

Some very simple, but important, steps can be taken to improve the quality of the foods consumed as part of a regular diet. They are:

- Eat organic foods as often as possible.

- Include a reasonable percentage of raw foods in your daily diet.

- Whenever possible, purchase foods from local growers.

- Purchase foods in season.

- Prepare meals from scratch using only natural and wholesome ingredients.

- Read the labels listing the ingredients contained in prepared foods and avoid those that have chemical additives, enhancers, and so on.

Eating Organically

There currently seems to be greater interest in and acceptance of organically grown foods. Unfortunately, a commonly expressed concern is its cost, as organic foods and natural products are more expensive than their highly processed and mass-produced counterparts. Over the years

I have come to see and appreciate the real value of that additional cost in the weekly budget. There are several reasons for this.

1. Organically grown food tastes like real food. Food certified organic is grown naturally without the use of chemical herbicides, pesticides, and artificial fertilizers. There are no chemical additives, flavorings, or food enhancers. According to law, only natural and wholesome ingredients can be used when an item is certified 100 percent organic.

2. Organic foods metabolize and are digested easily by the body. The liver, immune, and neurological systems are not compromised or impaired by such foods. The liver, especially, welcomes a reduced workload!

3. Organic foods are custom-made for organic bodies. The physical body welcomes the nutritional value and gains sustenance from the natural ingredients.

4. Organic foods fuel the body, providing energy that is needed for your physical body to perform optimally.

When the body is starved of essential nutrients, a natural response is to consume more food. This is an instinctual response by the body. In this regard, your body is giving you the message that additional nutrients are needed for healthy functioning. In some instances, being overweight is an indication of a body that is actually malnourished. In truth, your body will always let you know when something is out of balance internally, though you may not necessarily recognize this on a conscious level.

A well-balanced diet consisting mainly of organic foods will provide the basic nutrients for good health. Because of this, there is less need to consume large quantities of food. For the average household, the additional cost to the budget will, over time, be well worth it. My experience is that smaller servings of organic foods fill the nutritional void far better than larger servings of processed foods that are often devoid of nutritional benefits. There is also the additional benefit of improved physical health and increased energy levels, thereby saving costs on doctors' visits and medications.

There is considerable ongoing debate regarding the possible benefits of nutritional supplementation. Given the high level of toxins in the environment, I advocate taking daily nutritional supplements to assist the healthy functioning of the cellular, immune, and neurological systems. As awareness of the body's real needs increase (as cravings or habitual responses decrease), it becomes gradually easier to determine whether particular supplementation is needed or is beneficial. In other words, your body is perfectly capable of letting you know exactly what it needs to maintain health and well-being.

When changing to a diet comprising mainly organic foods, be prepared for some changes within the body. There is generally a period of adjustment, and even discomfort, that is experienced initially.

- When embarking on a natural food diet, you will find that practically all foods taste different. Fruits and vegetables taste real. Other organic foods, however, tend to taste less sweet, less salty, and less spicy. Foods seem bland, which means food will taste as it really is and not as it has been artificially created.

- Your body may experience withdrawal symptoms, as the common ingredients in processed foods are no longer being ingested. Sugar, fats, and food flavorings are commonplace in processed foods and their regular consumption results in cravings within the body. When they are no longer consumed, your body initially reacts as it does to the withdrawal of any substance it craves.

- Another initial change is that the body flushes out stored toxins that have accumulated over many years. It is quite common to experience headaches for a few days, to visit the bathroom more frequently, and to feel tired. There may even be skin eruptions, such as rashes or itching. All of this is perfectly normal and healthy. When this reaction occurs, accept that the body is expelling toxins and is not reacting to the newly introduced organic foods! My recommendation is to always ensure that there is an adequate intake of purified water, which assists the elimination process.

- As the body sheds the toxins and adjusts to the new diet of wholesome foods, there is an increased feeling of wellness, mental clarity, and renewed energy. There is also the likelihood of an improvement in metabolism.

- The immune system strengthens, decreasing susceptibility to viruses and a host of other contagious conditions.

- Over a period of time there will be obvious improvement in physical health as the body heals itself of any metabolic illnesses. There should be a noticeable improvement in health-related conditions such as diabetes, high blood pressure, cholesterol levels, arthritis, and heart disease, to mention only a few.

Enhancement of Protein Sources

It has become standard practice to modify fish, meat, and poultry that is available for public consumption. In theory, this makes the product more visually appealing to the consumer. In reality, any modification is intended to ensure plumper produce, so there is a greater yield from whatever beast or animal is being raised for human consumption. Color, antibiotics, and hormones are often included in the feed of protein food sources. Is it any wonder that many young girls enter puberty and begin their menses at a younger age than ever before? In recent years there have been reports about an increasing rate of infertility within the general population. The average semen count in males is reportedly decreasing.[17] What is the correlation between these phenomena and the standard practice of adding antibiotics and hormones into the food supply?

When eating protein foods that have been raised on pastures where no chemical herbicides, pesticides, and fertilizers have been used and without antibiotics or hormones added, there is a difference in the taste, texture, and color of the product. It is the same with fish that have not been modified in any way, but have been freshly caught in the wild. However, in the case of fish and seafood caught in areas close to ports

---

17. Sherril Sellman, ND. "The Problem of Precocious Puberty," *Nexus New Times* 19, no. 3. Deborah Cadbury. *Altering Eden: The Feminization of Nature*, St. Martin's Press, 1997.

and other industrial areas, there is always the added risk of mercury and other mineral and pollutant contamination. When changing to natural protein foods, less protein is needed with each serving, as it is nutrient rich and more easily metabolized and digested by the body.

Essential Enzymes

About thirty years ago, long before it became fashionable to eat a vegetarian diet, an acquaintance was forced to make drastic changes to her regular diet. Upon experiencing some confusing and obscure symptoms, she sought medical help. Eventually lupus was diagnosed. The prognosis for living a normal life seemed bleak. Numerous medications, including cortisone, were prescribed. Taking the medications created greater discomfort, so she began to read information on every natural option possible.

A book she read advocating a totally natural and raw food diet intrigued her. Luckily the author lived only a few hours away and so she arranged to visit him. As a result of that visit and his book, she is now slim, medication free, and living a normal, busy life. The reason for this is that her body began to heal when she embarked on a raw, natural food diet. It was not an easy process to adjust to; a great deal of the change involved trial and error—finding which foods were agreeable and which reacted in her body. However, she is a living example of how truly beneficial such a diet is for the human body.

I believe that making similar changes to the average diet would result in reducing the incidence of many illnesses. It is often said that around 60 percent of our daily food intake should be raw. This includes fruits, vegetables, seeds, and nuts. Research into enzyme functioning has shown that cooking destroys essential enzymes in food. This occurs when food is heated for twenty minutes at about 118 degrees Fahrenheit. Enzymes exist in raw food and play a critical role in breaking down foods in the digestive system.[18]

---

18. Edward Howell. *Enzyme Nutrition*, Avery Publishing, 1995.
     Mark Rojek. "The Essentials of Enzyme Nutrition Therapy," *Nexus New Times* 10, no. 6.

Energetic Impact

Improvements in health and well-being become evident in a relatively short period of time once an organic diet and the use of natural products are adopted. The physical body literally heals itself and thrives on such nourishment. The energy grid also thrives in these conditions. Organic foods, and especially raw and living food produce, energize the grid lines. These foods function as a natural fertilizer to the energy web that sustains life. Without chemicals and dead foods (denatured due to processing) in the diet, the energy grid is able to function as it was designed to function. The energy grid gradually restores its vitality, strength, and structure as the buildup of toxins is steadily released from the body.

Consumer Discernment

Supporting local growers is not only beneficial to the local economy, it also means that foods are fresher when purchased. Additionally, it affords an opportunity to find out exactly under what conditions the foods are grown, harvested, and processed. It does not take long to ask a few questions regarding the food about to be purchased in order to be sure you are purchasing good-quality foods. It is well known that there is a loss of nutritional value, especially vitamin C, in many fruits and vegetables within a relatively short time after harvesting. Local growers are able to harvest their crop and supply the community within a comparatively short time frame.

There is an increased tendency to find many more varieties of food produce readily available in supermarkets long after their growing season has ended. Fruits and vegetables purchased locally and in season are fresher and cheaper. Improved food technology has resulted in better storage and handling procedures for mass-produced foods. Yet we need to adhere to the principle of purchasing produce in season, thereby ensuring access to the freshest and most nutritionally beneficial foods.

Cooking Creatively

Consumers are rapidly losing the ability, time, and desire to create meals using only fresh and natural ingredients. Prepared meals and meal shortcuts are readily available in an ever-increasing abundance in supermarkets and are a great boon to the busy working family. They may often be a desirable and preferred option, especially after a long and hard day at work or school. However, it may be worth questioning what is actually contained in processed foods. Do they have residual toxins from chemicals used in food growing and processing? Are they the very best nutritional option for the body? In reality, it is far easier, more economical, and more beneficial for physical health to prepare a simple, nutritious meal using only natural ingredients.

Ultimately your body is the best indicator and barometer of what is most beneficial. When changing to a simpler, but no less delicious, natural and organic diet, the body enjoys the freedom from the many additives, chemicals, and unnatural flavors previously consumed. It especially enjoys the value of digesting nutritious foods instead of ingesting and having to process nutritionally empty foods that are often high in calories.

The more natural your diet, the more sensitized and in tune your body will become regarding what feels good when certain foods are eaten. Consequently, you will then be able to discern what foods do not agree with you, those that result in feelings of being bloated, uncomfortable, having headache reactions, and other symptoms, such as heartburn, indigestion, gastric ulcers, and so on.

Suggested Strategies

Take time to intimately discover what makes you feel well and what foods disagree with your body. This involves having greater mindfulness about what is placed in your mouth, as well as awareness of what is actually in the foods consumed.

- Simplify meals rather than overloading your digestive system with a mix of foods. Focus on using only one to three food groups in a meal. Prepare and cook these with a minimum of condiments and sauces.

- Eat less per serving. Be mindful of when you begin to feel full. Satiation occurs before the message registers in your consciousness. By fully focusing on each mouthful as you chew and by eating slower, you will begin to discern when fullness occurs.

- Observe and feel your body's reaction. Between meals drink water and abstain from continuous snacking. You will then be able to discern your body's response to the foods eaten.

- Shortly after they have been consumed, some foods will make you feel inordinately tired and even foggy in mental processing. Others may result in feelings of discomfort in the stomach; some may make you feel fidgety and restless. It may not necessarily be specific foods that trigger reactions, but rather ingredients that are found in a range of processed foods. For example, sugar, milk products, soy products, corn, wheat, and other fillers are commonly found in a large range of foods.

- Become adept at sensing what is happening within your body. It may be beneficial to keep a food journal in which you record what was eaten, the time of day, as well as any bodily reactions experienced. Over a period of a month, a noticeable pattern may be revealed.

This is a structured and practical way of determining how your body reacts to certain foods and ingredients. Armed with information on your body's reactions, you are then in a position to change or modify both diet and eating habits in order to heal your body.

Labeling Awareness

Read the labels on all food and personal care products you purchase. In practically all instances, they are confusing. The majority of the population does not have an understanding of biochemistry. There is little idea of what many of the listed ingredients actually mean and even less understanding of how they affect the molecular structure of cells, how they interact with other listed ingredients, and whether they accumulate within the fat cells and eventually damage DNA, cells, and organs.

In order to have a modicum of discernment in purchasing foods, I recommend buying a book from any bookstore or natural food outlet that stocks books on what is actually found in foods and personal care and household products. Take time to peruse and become familiar with at least some of the most commonly used chemical ingredients. There are far, far too many to memorize them all. When you find chemical ingredients listed on a product, search instead for an organic and chemical-free alternative.

It should be noted that there are a number of commonly used chemicals contained in personal care products that are damaging to the body and should definitely be avoided. The skin is by far the largest organ in the human body. Nerve cells are found close to the surface. The skin regulates perspiration, it breathes, and it is highly sensitive to toxins whether there is exposure through direct contact or from environmental fumes. It is important to ensure that what is applied topically is natural and nontoxic. Commonly used hair products, toothpaste, moisturizers, makeup, deodorants, shaving products, perfume, and so on contain a myriad of chemicals and alcohol that are detrimental to not only the skin but are absorbed into the body through the skin. Again, reading the labels and choosing to purchase products that contain nontoxic ingredients is integral to creating and sustaining good health. The benefits will become physically apparent in a matter of time.

Inhaling environmental pollutants is unavoidable. They are everywhere, but there are steps that can be taken to minimize exposure, especially in the home environment. Most household products contain hazardous chemicals, with many of them containing specific instructions on their handling. It is easy to become laissez faire when using them, not realizing that their poisons become stored in fat cells, in body tissue, and also have a damaging effect on organs, immune, and neurological systems. Nowadays, there are many organic, environmentally safe products available for home care. The short-term additional cost of purchasing natural products is well worth the long-term benefits to health.

There is another related aspect I wish to briefly draw your attention to. When purchasing organic and natural foods and products, you will be supporting a more traditional and natural way of farming and food production, which places less stress upon already depleted and over-worked mass-farmed soils. In choosing natural products, you will be healing not only your body but you will assist in healing the earth.

It is a matter of making a conscious decision to honor the body fully in all that you expose it to, whether internally or externally. Having that consciousness means taking the time and effort to become informed. This often means accessing information that is not necessarily readily available in the popular media. Consciously question the media's role through advertising in promoting certain products, lifestyle, and beliefs. Be aware that much of what you believe about your body and your eating and lifestyle habits are the result of great marketing and advertising campaigns.

Remember the story I shared about my acquaintance with lupus? By choosing to seek, to question, and to believe she was entitled to have not only a healthy body but also a quality lifestyle, she was able to make conscious and informed choices around her diet and lifestyle that have since proved fruitful. Her story epitomizes the wisdom contained in the saying "Let food be our medicine, and our medicine be our food"!

- Have an awareness of what foods and lifestyle products you place in your shopping cart.
- Be mindful of the impact they will likely have on your body.
- If they contain chemicals, you have the right to ask for and expect a natural alternative.
- Honor your body at all times—buy only what promotes health and well being.
- As you begin making changes in your purchasing power, view it as a process and take it one step at a time.
- The more you undertake this process, the more you will attract new information and experiences that will remind you of its value and ultimate benefits.

You begin by making meaningful changes for yourself, and from there you will progress to sharing with family and friends the reasons for making such changes. Consumer purchasing power is extremely powerful. Demand and expect only food and products that are contaminant-free. The greater the demand for natural foods and products, the more that will be produced to meet that demand.

Creating a healthy body begins with you. Choosing foods and products that support and nourish you daily are an integral and essential component of creating healing and wellness on the physical level.

CHAPTER TEN

Sleep: For Body and Soul

"If you are at peace with yourself,
you will discern peace around you."
—*Sri Sathya Sai Baba*—

A recent television advertisement claimed that more than one million Americans regularly have difficulty sleeping. My immediate thought was that while this is a considerable portion of the population, perhaps the figure is actually greater than this. Clients often share that they've come to need less sleep as they age and consider it a normal consequence of aging. Modern living is becoming increasingly complex. Relentless and conflicting demands are most likely training your body to survive and function with less sleep. That does not mean you need less sleep or rest. In fact, most people I speak with, whether in a professional capacity or socially, comment that they continually feel tired. This tiredness can be attributed to many factors, including lifestyle and beliefs.

Social conditioning deems that the average person functions according to the demands of time. In most Western households the day begins with the ringing of the alarm clock. This does not necessarily mean that your body is ready to awaken. Once awake, and in many instances not fully awake but attempting to function as if you are, the day begins. The average day is filled with organized activities that are often time determined. Rushing from one appointment to the next is commonplace. It is normal to schedule the days so fully that often it is not possible to stop until well after sundown. Most people then wonder why there is no reservoir of energy, and consequently the familiar couch and television look enticing.

Culturally it has become acceptable to believe that each and every minute of the day needs to be gainfully occupied. Incessant busyness, being productive, taking an interest in the external world, and ensuring that not a minute is wasted is highly valued and socially encouraged. It is normal to be constantly physically engrossed and mentally involved in a range of issues.

What is the conditioning that has created the belief that life has to be lived at a frenetic pace? Working to survive is a basic tenet for most people. The need to earn income is unavoidable, though this now seems to be the main priority, or *raison d'être*, for a large portion of the population. Indigenous cultures never faced this dilemma. Their days were balanced with a number of activities, including hunting, gathering, creating, working communally, and devoting time to spiritual practice. It seems the luxury of living such a balanced life is no longer a viable option for the population at large. Instead, a belief system around the importance of achieving financial security has been indoctrinated and is now firmly entrenched in cultural mores. A system has been created in which it is impossible to survive without financial assets. Simultaneously, great emphasis is placed upon the need to continually purchase and upgrade belongings. A system of bondage has been established—a system that lacks balance and that places considerable stress upon most people.

It is commonly accepted that it is normal to be fully occupied for every minute of the day. How often do you find an unexpected spare time slot in your day or week only to immediately look to how best to fill that void? Perhaps idleness is to be avoided at all costs? Maybe, at a subconscious level, idleness is viewed as sinful. Or maybe conditioning reinforces the belief that busyness is productive and achievement-oriented, and these are considered highly desirable traits. By continually striving to keep busy, it becomes difficult to stop.

An acquaintance contracted mononucleosis, which necessitated two months' absence from work. She was ambitious and was continually involved in numerous activities as well as being career-oriented. Her lifestyle created substantial internal stress, and the illness enforced a period of rest. There was no option but to relax, and she gainfully used the rest to learn what was happening in her body. After a great deal of soul searching, she eventually came to view her body as a marvelous piece of machinery that had collapsed from exhaustion in order to rebuild itself. Consequently she learned to feel, observe, and listen to the body's messages and eventually came to an understanding of its needs. She learned to be more in tune with her unique machinery!

The human body is like a vehicle. When it is only driven in top gear, its potential performance is greatly undermined. It is easy to forget to wind up slowly in the morning. Starting from neutral gear and immediately shifting to overdrive is fairly common practice. Most people omit the gears in between. These gears help minimize stress and are designed to gradually and gracefully allow for the build up of greater and therefore less stressful momentum to the day.

In order to add improved acceleration to the average daily start-up, a turbo-charged, caffeine-laden coffee is added first thing every morning. Often a single turbo-charge is insufficient for full momentum, and so by lunchtime several cups of coffee are needed to sustain energy levels. Over time, a rushed start to the day has a damaging and stressful effect on the body. The use of stimulants to maintain functioning in top gear is detrimental and eventually creates specific problems, including adrenal burnout.[19]

Mental and emotional confusion and fear add to daily stresses. It is easy to carry considerable chatter and clutter in the mind, so it is no wonder anxiety and worry become constant companions. Imagine how difficult it must be for the physical body to relax sufficiently and get a good night's sleep when the internal chatter is relentless.

Clients have shared that one of the most common effects of an energy healing session is extreme tiredness within twenty-four hours of having the session. My immediate response is to ask that they honor that tiredness, take a nap, and allow a longer than usual sleep at night. During sleep, cells regenerate and the body heals itself. Instinctively the body knows exactly what it needs and also knows how to do it. However, it is normal to hold a great deal of stress in the body. This stress is due to lifestyle, diet, and thoughts that interfere with the body's natural sleep pattern.

The scientific study of sleep patterns has revealed that the body goes through a number of sleep phases, each of them important and essential for healing. The last phase of deep sleep occurs naturally just before you awaken. If your alarm is continually set to an early hour, it is most likely that this critical sleep phase is missed. Sleep deprivation then sets in, accumulates over time, and eventually affects general health.

There is an abundance of literature on how to ensure a good night's sleep. In order to have deep and healing sleep, it is important to reduce the amount of stress within the body. I have been guided to follow a few simple strategies and these may be helpful.

---

19. Jesse Lynn Hanley, MD, and Nancy Deville. *Tired of Being Tired*, Berkley Publishing Group, 2001.

Suggested Strategies

- Eat lightly for the evening meal and allow a minimum of three hours between eating and going to sleep. This means there is less digestive processing during sleep, thereby enabling the body to relax and heal. Digestion is a process—it requires energy and places additional stress on the organs and the nervous and digestive systems.

- Following a food-combining diet assists digestion and is less stressful on the body. Different foods require different digestion and assimilation time. When studied extensively, it becomes apparent that food-combining can be a complex process. Needless to say, there are some simple guidelines that can be adhered to. For example, fruit should always be eaten on an empty stomach as it moves rapidly through the digestive system. Proteins should not be consumed with starches and grains; they should be eaten at seperate meals. If you suffer from indigestion regularly, it may be worthwile to explore food-combining priniples.[20]

- Eliminating caffeine, alcohol, and nicotine helps significantly. The damaging effects of all three on the body have been amply researched. My guidance from other dimensions have reiterated the importance of eliminating these because of their deleterious impact upon the sensitive energy grid. If you are unable or unwilling to eliminate caffeine, alcohol, or nicotine from your lifestyle, at least minimize consumption. Endeavor to abstain from mid-afternoon on, as this will enable your body to rid itself from the effects of whatever you have inhaled or ingested.

- Incorporate regular exercise into your daily routine. A physical workout during the day has a multitude of benefits. Your body sleeps better after physical activity.

---

20. Alissa Cohen. *Living on Live Food*, Cohen Publishing Co., 2004. www.healingdaily.com/detoxification-diet/food-combining.com www.thewolfeclinic.com/foodcombining.html http://weightloss.about.com/cs/foodcombining/.

- Allow the body to relax and wind down prior to sleep. Television is often used as a means of providing that relaxation. It cannot be relaxing to a body already overloaded by toxins and stress to be subjected to suspenseful drama, action, noise, and violence as is often depicted on a great number of nightly televised programs. Activities that quiet the mind are advisable. They include reading for pleasure and not for business or study purposes, hobbies, meditation, and listening to quiet, soothing music.

- Create a relaxing environment. There seems to be a trend occurring where many homes now have a television set in each bedroom. The effects of continual exposure to electromagnetic frequencies on the body are only now becoming widely known. I have read literature recommending that absolutely no electrical appliances should be located in the bedroom. The reason for this is that electromagnetic frequencies from electrical appliances create interference within the body's natural energy field, over time depleting it and resulting in ill health. Your sleep state is a time for the body to rest and self-heal; electromagnetic frequencies interfere with this critical process.

My spiritual guidance has stressed the importance of reducing the amount of time spent working with and being around electronic equipment, as their charges and frequencies disturb the natural energy field. Endless hours spent watching television and playing and working with computer technology all interfere greatly. I have been told that they dim the energy field, dull the senses, weaken the immune system, increase susceptibility to illness and disease, and affect mental acuity and functioning. In fact, the antidote to electromagnetic frequency overload is to spend time in the natural environment where the energy balance in the body has a chance to become restored and whole again.

- Regular bodywork sessions, including massage, assist in releasing pent-up stress and stored emotions. Yoga, Pilates, and other exercises involving deep and relaxed breathing are also recommended. Activities such as these facilitate inner harmony and balance within the body and are a wonderful means of reducing stress.

- Assess the perceptions you hold about sleep. When you say and believe that going to sleep is difficult, then that is what happens. Instead, affirm that your body is going to have a sound night's sleep and then continue thinking this. In time your body will respond to that message, and you will find that this mental preparation, along with some of the other strategies suggested, will ensure your body is receiving adequate rest.

There are also times when your body requires additional rest in order to maintain vitality and energy levels. In learning to heed your body's messages, you will come to know when rest is necessary, and not merely desirable. In many Mediterranean cultures siesta is practiced, where resting in the mid-afternoon is normal. Surely there must be some real and lasting benefits to this tradition.

In a message received from my spiritual guidance several years ago, it became evident that sitting and doing absolutely nothing is never a waste of time. Apparently the cells in the body regenerate completely every seven years. To my way of thinking it is preferable to give support and assistance to this regeneration process. Cells have a way of mutating and multiplying unnaturally when certain conditions exist within the body. In honoring the body by listening to its messages and heeding its needs, there is a likelihood you can live your life productively and healthily into old age.

Energetic Implications

Sleep is essential for physical, mental, and emotional functioning. Whatever happens on the physical level is affected by your mental and emotional states, and vice versa. The three are inescapably interlinked. When sleep deprivation occurs, the physical body functions below par. Similarly, your mental and emotional faculties are also impaired. Mental processing becomes faulty, resulting in a lack of clarity and possibly accuracy. Emotional responses tend to be intense and may even become irrational. Ultimately, the quality of life is affected on every level when sleep needs are not met. The end result is a state of imbalance on the physical, mental, and emotional levels. The impact is also experienced in the energy field as the stress takes its toll on the sensitive energy grids, resulting in gridlines that become weakened and out of alignment.

During sleep, cells repair and regenerate. Similarly, the energy grid undertakes its repair and regeneration. All living matter undertakes this process in some form, though the cycles obviously vary. For humans the circadian cycle has distinct phases, and time for rest and sleep is one of these. This time is cleverly built in so that self-healing can occur within the body and on all levels. It is during this time that your exposure to multiple stresses, emotions, and toxins is reduced.

On another level, sleep is an opportunity for your inner essence, or soul, to surface. During the day, while your conscious mind is busily dealing with daily demands, there is often little or no opportunity for your soul to make its presence or needs felt. While in sleep, your conscious mind also closes down, and it is then that your soul is able to deliver its messages. These may come in the form of lucid dreams and astral traveling. Sometimes they are delivered in a specific way so that when you awaken you have a strong knowing or desire to take a certain course of action. It is in the first few minutes of consciousness, before fully awakening, that the knowing surfaces. This knowing comes from deep within and reveals itself before the reality and distractions of another day intrude. These thoughts are a form of communication from your soul.

Having a good night's sleep is as important to your overall health, healing, and well-being as eating organic and natural foods. Each plays a critical role in ensuring a balanced body on all levels. Without either, imbalance occurs on some level, and the resultant distress to the body eventually becomes evident. In the following chapter I will explore what is actually meant by being in balance and how to create it, primarily, on a physical level. Later chapters will focus more on the mental, emotional, and spiritual levels and what is needed to create balance in those areas.

CHAPTER ELEVEN
Balance in All Things

"The most wasted of all days is that
on which one has not laughed."
—Nicolas Chamfort—

"Remember to have balance in all things," my spiritual guidance often says. Where there is balance, there is inner harmony. A balanced energy field means equilibrium of the mental, physical, emotional, and spiritual levels. Focusing primarily on one of these levels results in an imbalance within the energy field, thereby creating a similar state in an individual's life. There are people who are highly focused and driven, whether it is in regard to their spiritual path, their chosen career, or some other interest. This obvious passion, which may produce outstanding results in a specific area, often results in disregard and neglect of other equally important aspects of life. As an example, it is easy to overlook the need for recreation pursuits and regular exercise to maintain the body's flexibility and healthy functioning, especially as competing demands take priority. You have incarnated to learn and practice integrating the physical, mental, emotional, and spiritual levels into one harmonious and unified body. When allowing your body to be out of balance without endeavoring to restore its natural harmony, you are giving it a literal message that you do not consider it important.

Balance on the physical level involves healthy eating, having good sleep patterns, and undertaking regular exercise. A balanced body is reflected in good health and the ability to cope with the stresses and demands of daily life. Emotional balance involves being in a state of calmness and acceptance. It means that emotions do not control your responses. Instead, you are able to manage your emotions. Mental balance can be explained as having clarity of mental processing and not reacting irrationally. When continual thinking and worry dominate every waking moment, this could signal an imbalance on the mental level. This is not the same as having a mental illness. Because we live in a world that is constantly changing and we are exposed to a wide range of stresses, maintaining balance on all levels is a continuous process and involves awareness of the subtleties that create balance and those that result in disharmony.

Your body continually sends messages so that changes necessary for optimal functioning can be made. Similarly, your body constantly receives messages from you regarding your perception of life. These messages have an impact upon the body that in time manifests to create the beliefs you communicate. This may seem to be a catch-22 situation. One affects the other. The two are intermeshed and interlinked. Ultimately, whatever you give out is what you get back. It is erroneous to think this principle applies mainly to interactions with family, friends, colleagues, and so on. This is a universal law and applies to everything.

Recreation

Recreation and exercise are essential to good health. Yet, how often are these neglected when the demands of work and family intrude? The truism, "Use it or lose it," applies in this instance. Hectic schedules often limit the time available for such pursuits, and television viewing generally ends up being both the recreation and exercise routine for many people.

Recreational activities are generally set aside for any spare time that is left at the end of the working day or week. It is usual to seek out and engage in activities that are enjoyable, creative, and fun. However, it is all too easy to put your need for these last, especially when there are many competing priorities. It has been my experience that when this aspect is neglected I end up feeling incomplete and eventually resentful of other competing priorities. It is a familiar story that is also shared by friends, clients, and participants in the workshops I conduct. By scheduling recreational activity as a regular routine, there inevitably is a feeling of balance, satisfaction, and enjoyment incorporated into life.

The working world tends to be goal-focused and achievement-oriented. It is very easy to allow work to become all-consuming and engrossing. Often I hear of people who have had highly successful working lives and then found themselves at a loss when retirement occurs. Recreation offers an opportunity to creatively explore and develop aspects of your capabilities and interests that otherwise would remain dormant. Many of these have the potential to be utilized meaningfully upon retirement.

Again and again I encounter people who are dissatisfied with their career choices. They indicate that they just happened to choose a certain profession and have felt bound to it, mainly because of employment security and the added benefits. It is sad to think that sometimes people spend more than a third of their lives working in a field that is not satisfying or lacking enjoyment. The stresses of being in such a situation must be overwhelming. When this is the case there is all the more reason for creating a balance of activities into the weekly schedule. In these instances both recreational pursuits and a regular exercise regime help inordinately in easing the stresses created as a result of feeling trapped in a particular career option.

Essential Exercise

The benefits of regular exercise have been expounded time and again, and a proportion of the population engages in some form of activity beneficial to their health. Regular exercise is critical to healthy functioning. It assists metabolism and oxygenation of the blood, ensures muscular strength and flexibility, increases resistance to disease, and so on. Best of all, it is a great endorphin releaser, thereby enhancing feelings of well-being.

Surprisingly, regular exercise actually increases energy levels. It enables you to think more clearly and concisely, as well as giving your body the stamina needed for daily activities. Often, at the end of a long and challenging day, physical activity is least desired. However, even a short twenty-minute walk around the neighborhood delivers surprising benefits. Your body is designed to be ambulatory and physically active. It is not designed for hours of sitting, thereby placing considerable strain on the spinal column, organs, and digestive system.

Theories and ideas abound as to what is creating the increasing levels of obesity in the general population. Perhaps a significant contributing factor may be that generally people are more sedentary. It is no longer necessary to work as physically hard as earlier generations. In those times, hard physical work ensured survival. Nowadays there is motorized transport and technological conveniences for all needs.

Without regular exercise the body atrophies, muscles become wasted, and gradual signs of vitality loss are exhibited. Compare the obvious signs of vitality emanating from an athlete or someone who regularly exercises with someone who avoids exercise. The first noticiable thing is skin health. Exercisers look hale and exude energy. Their skin has a healthy glow. The skin of non-exercisers over time begins to look insipid and lax. Regular moderate exercise lubricates the body and ensures its healthy functioning.

Breath Invigorates

Underpinning the value of undertaking regular exercise is the importance of breath, or *Prana*, which is your life force. When undertaking regular exercise, correct breathing becomes critical to optimal functioning. With deep breathing, the oxygen circulates throughout the whole body, sustaining and nourishing it. In my healing practice I see many people who do not breathe properly. Their breath is shallow, going no deeper than the thoracic cavity. They wonder why their bodies are sore and holding a lot of stress. Correct breathing is deep breathing and involves inhaling right into the lower abdominal region. Most people when taught this procedure say it feels strange, which it does if they've not previously learned how to breathe deeply and slowly, but after a while it becomes second nature. With regular deep breathing, blood is able to circulate freely, as it is not starved for oxygen. With this, nutrients are also better filtered to cells for healthy growth and body wastes better circulated for elimination.

Natural deep breathing is also wonderful for releasing stress. After a stressful and commitment-packed day, an evening walk is a remarkable tonic. The stored stress can be released consciously. Whatever has contributed to the stress, frustration, and maybe even anger is brought forward to the conscious mind. On each breath inhalation, focus on bringing in clean revitalizing energy, which is then breathed deep into the lower abdominal region. The exhalation releases all the murkiness of the stress and any negative emotions that have been stored. This simple exercise literally breathes out and releases stored emotions. By the time you return home you will feel calmer and clearer within. This process is a healthy and painless way of removing negative emotions almost as soon as they occur, and even more so, it prevents their festering within the body.

I cannot stress enough the importance of correct breathing at all times. It is easy to take your breathing for granted, thereby losing awareness of it within your body. Yoga practitioners and those who study ancient Eastern practices know only too well how essential it is to every aspect of well-being. If people learned to breathe as their bodies are designed for, many indeterminate conditions and discomforts within the body would be a thing of the past.

Having consciousness of breathing habits and patterns can be very revealing. Do you at times almost forget to breathe as you become engrossed in some activity? Or is your breathing almost always shallow and rapid? In order to create good health, the breath should always be relaxed, deep, and gentle. Once you have an awareness of your breath patterns, consciously endeavor to spend about five to ten minutes a day practicing deeper breathing. It will seem strange at first, almost as though it is forced, and may even feel tiring. Perseverance will pay off and, as with all new learning, will in time integrate, soften, and feel normal. As you begin to consciously undertake this exercise, be mindful of the state of your body. Is it feeling stressed? Can you feel a fluttering of inner nervous tension? If so, be aware of how your body feels as you focus on your breathing. It should begin to relax, tension should dissipate, and your mind will also begin to calm.

Bodywork Benefits

Another way of assisting the body to release stored tension is to engage in regular bodywork sessions. Massage is probably the most commonly known and accepted of these. The mere act of regularly relaxing for an hour or more while entrusting the body to a qualified therapist is not an indulgence. It is an integral component of the self-healing journey. Skilled therapists, whether massage or other healing modalities, are able to assist the body to release stored tension, balance the body's energies, and facilitate the body's natural self-healing mechanisms. When the physical body is treated to a bodywork session, healing takes place on many levels, not solely the physical level. The emotional, mental, and spiritual levels also benefit greatly.

In my practice I often see clients who address their self-healing mainly through mind or intellectual activities, including psychotherapy and meditation. They then wonder why their physical body suffers from various ailments, often minor but nevertheless disconcerting and inconvenient to their lifestyle. The healing of many physical symptoms experienced by most of the population can be achieved through regular bodywork sessions. Some bodywork options include massage, chiropractic, acupuncture, osteopathy, Bowen, and reflexology.

Regular bodywork not only supports the healing process, but it can also be used as a vital ingredient in a wellness maintenance program. It is easy to focus energies only on regaining health and well-being when one or more ailments are experienced. It is far better to maintain sound health, high energy levels, and general well-being than having to deal with symptoms and causes of ill health. Regular bodywork sessions play a valuable role in preventive medicine and wellness maintenance!

In most instances, a family pattern of health conditions may be traced back through several generations, for example, high blood pressure, heart conditions, and cancer. When this is the case, every endeavor to prevent ill health should be integrated into a holistic wellness program. Keep in mind that allopathic medicine focuses on dealing with the condition once it makes its presence known. Holistic therapies incorporate practices to enhance well-being and sound health. It is far better (and cheaper) to prevent heart illness or any other condition than it is to seek a cure after its onset!

Environmental Healing

It is interesting to observe the increasing trend in the general population toward spending time in the natural environment. Many people walk, jog, and spend time undertaking recreational pursuits in nature's greenery. My first reaction when entering a natural forest is to deeply inhale the rich oxygen source given off by plant life. My body feels like it is receiving an "instant hit" of life-giving energy, which is what actually occurs.

The human body has had to adjust to urban living and is exposed daily to pollution, environmental toxins, and population congestion. The body actually thrives in an environment that is the exact opposite. Anyone who has a love of nature and spending time outdoors understands precisely what I'm referring to. My spiritual teaching has consistently revolved around the benefits of reconnecting with Mother Nature and of the value to the human body when time is spent in her energies.

Taking time out from the hectic demands of daily living and reconnecting with natural energies is a wonderful restorative. It is one of the most healing ways to spend recreation and exercise time. Traditional cultures lived in harmony with the natural environment. They learned from it, respected its power and energy, and through this came to great understanding and acceptance of the nature of cycles.

You are closely linked to everything through energy because you are energy. Whatever happens in nature affects you and vice versa—everything is interlinked and interconnected. Connecting with the energy of nature through your activities, whether they are strenuous or leisurely, creates awareness of this connection, however subtle it may be. When the intention of compassion and peace is brought into the natural environment, this is immediately sensed by the natural habitat. The opposite applies too, as negative emotions are also easily sensed. Your interactions with nature are similar to the intuitive response experienced when you initially meet someone. The energy you hold is sensed, and immediately there is a reaction within the natural habitat.

Whatever happens in our lives, as a community and globally, is reflected in the state of the natural environment. Mother Earth is a mirror for all emotions and actions. If a state of cooperation and global peace existed, there would not be the extent of natural disasters and environmental catastrophes currently occurring. The environmental chaos is a reflection of the inner chaos experienced within humanity.

In this chapter, five areas that are essential and critical to any process of self-healing have been briefly explored. The reason for this brevity is that there is ample information available elsewhere on strategies and application of these principles. Recreation, exercise, correct breathing, having regular bodywork sessions, and connecting with the natural environment are essential to any self-healing process. Their practice enriches the energy field due to the feelings of wellness experienced. As you begin to self-heal on all levels, you will find changes occurring in people close to you, as well as within your general environment. Self-healing does not take place in a cocoon and is not a solitary experience. Nor is substantial healing possible when you rely totally on other people and external sources. In order to achieve self-healing, an inner journey of exploration and discovery is necessary for real improvements to occur.

The following chapters will cover (in greater depth) aspects of the inner journey process. Simple steps will be advocated to enhance progress and growth. As with all things, there is one important element to be aware of and that is trust. When you trust that changes and growth are inevitable and that everything will unfold for your highest good, that is exactly what happens. Once you embark upon this journey, there can be no turning back, regardless of how challenging the journey may be at times. The rewards in terms of inner peace and improvement in physical health are well worth the journey!

Energy Infusion (refer to CD)

This exercise allows you to focus energy during breath work and, when practiced regularly, will assist you in creating additional energy abundance for daily needs. It also enhances feelings of inner calm and balance.

Sit comfortably wherever you choose. Keep your back straight, your legs uncrossed, and your feet on the floor. Rest your arms gently on your lap. Breathe in deeply and slowly. Exhale gently. Repeat this breath cycle a few times. Feel your body gradually relaxing. As your breath circulates freely, feel the stored tension releasing from every part of your body.

On your next inhalation, visualize your breath reaching into every cell of your body. Feel it flowing into the very tips of your fingers and toes. Hold your breath for a count of four and then gently exhale. As you exhale, visualize the exhalation releasing your stresses and emotions. Repeat this process several times until you feel totally relaxed and energized by your oxygen-rich breath.

As you continue circulating the enriching and sustaining energy of your breath, visualize yourself surrounded by white light. Breathe in this white light. Breathe it into every cell, every atom, and every molecule of your body. Feel your body slowly and steadily absorbing the white light. You are becoming a brilliant orb of white light. Feel the flow of the white light as it moves through your body, from your head to your feet.

See the light flowing out of your feet and upward, totally filling your physical body and your energy field. As the white light reaches the top of your head, feel it being absorbed into your physical body once again. Feel the continuing circular flow of light energy as it flows through your physical body, into your energy field, and back into your physical body.

Now direct your attention to your feet. They are sitting in a glowing pool of red light. This is earth energy. It is strong and balanced. Feel this red light moving slowly through your feet, up your legs, and through your body, until it spills up out of your crown like a fountain and down through your energy field. Feel the stabilizing and healing power of the earth as your energy field is filled with red glowing light.

Glowing white and red light is now circulating freely within you and through you. Allow this light to flow through your body and energy field several times until your body is ablaze with light. The light moves freely and eliminates all stress and tension from your mind, body, and spirit, leading you to complete inner calm and balance. Know that you have sufficient energy for your day's needs. The relaxed and calm feelings will remain with you throughout the day. When you are ready, bring your awareness back into the room where you are sitting.

Earth Energy

This simple and brief exercise will assist you to feel the energies in nature and will, with practice, enable you to connect energetically with trees, plants, and the earth. Connecting energetically with the environment is healthy for the energy grid as it assists its healing and restoration of the energetic balance.

Find a place in the natural environment, facing about 24 inches from a large tree, and stand comfortably in a relaxed manner. You may wish to close your eyes, as this will assist your focus. Feel your breath as it goes through your body. Then feel your whole body. Feel the energies flowing within your body.

Lift your arms from the elbow, with palms facing outward. Slowly move them forward toward the tree but without touching it. Stop moving when you feel a slight resistance. You are now connecting with the energy from the tree. Softly, in your mind, ask for permission to share the tree's energy. Intuitively, you will sense its positive response.

Slowly move your body forward toward the tree. The aim is to experience the full energy of the tree in your energy field, not just what is felt in your hands. You may feel tingling sensations within your body during this sharing of energies. The tree is an active participant in the energy sharing! When finished, silently thank the tree.

This is only one method of connecting with nature. As you become familiar with the energy of trees, you may wish to stand further back, open your heart center, and ask that the tree feel your heart energy. In time you will be able to stand several feet away and draw the energy of a tree into your energy field, while simultaneously expanding your energy so that the tree experiences your beautiful energy.

Similarly, it will become relatively easy to feel the energy of Mother Earth. When standing in a relaxed manner, feel her energies surging up through your feet and into your body. These energies circulate and revitalize your energies.

CHAPTER TWELVE
Meditation Magic

"Inner harmony is your greatest supporter
in bearing the burden of life."
—Paramahansa Yogananda—

Several years ago a Buddhist nun gave an inspiring talk in Perth, Western Australia. Tenzin Palmo was born in Britain and at a relatively young age had traveled to India to learn more about the meaning of life. After studying with a number of masters, Tenzin Palmo eventually came to the realization that if she really wanted to know more she needed to isolate herself in order to find the answers that lay within. This she did by retreating to a cave in the Himalayan Mountains.

During her twelve-year retreat she grew vegetables in a small area outside her cave and also received regular supplies of provisions from nearby villagers when weather conditions were favorable. She recounted her experiences of the harsh winters. At one stage she became quite ill and had to fend for herself, as she didn't have the luxury of being able to visit a nearby doctor. The account of her odyssey is shared in the book *Cave In The Snow*.[21] During her talk she offered profound insights, and I will now share one of these.

Tenzin Palmo reminded the audience that Western society focuses interest and intent on material acquisition and possessions. Great joy and pride are taken in whatever is acquired. Being proud homeowners, it is common to perform ongoing cleaning and maintenance of the home. She highlighted the fact that a great deal of satisfaction is derived in thoroughly spring-cleaning the home or highly prized car. In much the same manner, from time to time the physical body receives additional care. This may involve an intestinal or liver cleanse, a weight-loss program, some form of cosmetic enhancement, or purchasing a new wardrobe.

However, while continually seeking to improve many aspects of life, there is a tendency to overlook giving the mind a regular and much needed spring-clean. The mind, like household closets, tends to become cluttered over time. The average mind becomes filled with chatter and outdated beliefs and perceptions, and for some reason this is deemed acceptable and normal. Ironically, while most people accept this as the status quo, they simultaneously complain that it is impossible to gain respite from the endless chatter! From this analogy Tenzin Palmo then

21.   Vicki Mackenzie. *Cave In the Snow,* Bloomsbury, 1998.

shared with the audience why meditation is so important; she described its numerous benefits and also why it can be practiced by anyone. Meditation does not have to be complicated or difficult, and the more it is practiced, the more its benefits become evident.

Often I reflect on her analogy of the cluttered mind and its need for regular doses of spring-cleaning. It is common to hear clients complain about the fact that their mind never stops due to constant worry. The chatter is endless and relentless. It is not a comfortable position to be in and is cause for considerable aggravation and annoyance for many people. My spiritual guides have been consistent with their message regarding the importance of making time for daily reflection or meditation. Often, lack of time is viewed as a major limitation to undertaking regular meditative practice. In reality, you make time for the necessities of daily living. Daily ablutions, an exercise program, and anything else considered vitally important are slotted into your schedule. Given the fact that most people ensure time is devoted to worthy and necessary habits, I have been assured by those from another dimension that including regular meditation practice is essential to physiological, psychological, and spiritual growth and awareness.

Devoting anywhere from a few minutes to up to an hour daily will result in improvement in all facets of life. Meditation is a wonderful tool for assisting the individual to go within, to find the answers to many of life's challenges, and to aid in the awakening of the spiritual self. An obvious benefit of meditation is relaxation. For those whose lives and minds are continually abuzz with all sorts of worry, concerns, and challenges, regularly devoting a few minutes to meditation will assist in giving greater peace of mind and clarity of thought. Daily meditation invariably helps you function better.

During meditation your body is stilled on all levels. A state of suspension exists. This state is beneficial to the energy grid because in this suspended state, the golden balls of energy become energized. This results in a charge being produced, which is then transmitted to the fine silken threads. Consequently the silken threads are given a boost of healing from receiving this subtle energy charge.

Brain Wave Functioning

When an EEG (electroencephalograph or brain wave scan) is performed on meditators, there is a greater state of alpha waves. Alpha waves also occur during one of the light sleep or dreaming patterns experienced when sleeping. The alpha wave is relaxing, almost placing the individual into an altered state of consciousness. Becoming adept at meditation results in considerable change to the natural brain wave pulsing. Alpha states enable you to access inner creativity and lead to deeper states of consciousness. They have been found to support inner calmness, alertness, deeper knowing and learning as well as enhanced mental coordination.

Interestingly, the study of brain waves only commenced in the early twentieth century. Brain wave research has focused on meditation, hypnotherapy, biofeedback, and neurology. Alpha waves are the most well-known and easily identified of all the brain waves, with a frequency varying from 7–8Hz to 12Hz, depending upon the individual. The average value of alpha waves is 10.5Hz. Another two rhythm signals involved in meditative states are the theta and delta waves. On an EEG, they are identifiable below the 8Hz frequencies.

Theta waves (4–7Hz), while occurring mainly in sleep, are also evident in deep states of meditation. In this state the senses have escaped from the external reality and are totally focused on the inner landscape. In a theta state you become receptive to information that is normally outside your external sensory awareness. Meditation in this state reduces stress, enhances creativity, and increases intuition and extrasensory perception. Delta waves (0–4Hz) are the slowest of the brain waves. These occur in dreamless sleep and in the deepest of meditation states. When meditating at this frequency, there are profound feelings of peace and calmness and a total suspension of the external reality.[22]

---

22. R. A. Miller and I. Miller. "The Schumann's Resonances and Human Psychobiology," *Nexus New Times* 10, no. 3.

Benefits

The practice of regular meditation results in improvement of many physiological conditions. Scientific evidence now proves it is instrumental in reducing elevated blood pressure and relieving pain and stress. Conditions that benefit from regular meditation practice include: substance addiction, fibromyalgia, asthma, irritable bowel syndrome, ulcers, insomnia, cancer, AIDS, auto-immune diseases, heart disease, infertility, premenstrual tension, psoriasis, and tension headaches. If for any reason you are experiencing a condition of ill health, there is every indication that incorporating meditation into your self-healing regime will gradually reap benefits.

Psychological benefits abound from regular meditation practice. It is useful in healing old traumas, forgiveness issues, confronting death, dealing with wellness anxieties, and enhancing self-esteem. Those who have been practicing meditation for a long time and experience deep meditations have increased activity in the left prefrontal cortex. When people are in a state of happiness, this area is active. Depression is associated with right prefrontal dominance. Meditation works on increasing the happiness levels and could even be considered to have antidepressant benefits!

Why Meditate?

Diverse cultures and peoples around the world have used meditation for healing and as part of traditional religious practice for thousands of years. The value of meditation to alleviate suffering and promote healing is well known and accepted within many traditions.

Often learning meditation techniques is resorted to when there are no other options available for dealing with stress. This is common in clients who are seeking some means of assuaging whatever pain they are experiencing. A woman had enormous work-related stresses that resulted in both physical and emotional pain. Her instinctual solution to the problem was to learn meditation and to use it as a means of being able to cope with the nonstop conflicts and high-pressure demands in the workplace. Interestingly, it was not long before she noticed a significant change in working conditions. Nothing had actually changed except her perception and way of dealing with situations as they arose. She also found herself becoming more assertive and clear about her level of responsibility in ensuring her well-being at all times.

There is no denying that a regular exercise program is essential to the management of stress and for overall well-being. However, the additional inclusion of regular meditation practice assists enormously. Meditation clears and calms the mind, and in the process allows for greater creativity, resourcefulness, and the ability to manage stress in a meaningful way. This means that constant stress is no longer a dominant factor in decision-making. Meditation assists you to take back control of whatever occurs in your life.

It has been my experience that when meditating for a specific reason, for example, emotional trauma, meditation facilitates the release of blocked energies around that trauma while simultaneously effecting changes on the physical and mental levels. In releasing the emotions around the trauma, there will be less mind chatter around the pain, resulting in greater clarity of thought. The physical body happily welcomes the release of the emotional trauma, feels lighter, and has more energy to expend.

There is a commonly held expectation that great insights and significant inner changes will be achieved within a relatively short space of time. Meditation, irrespective of the technique used, takes time to master. In much the same way, it takes a period of time for results to become evident when undergoing a weight-loss and fitness regime. A minimum of six to eight weeks is often the time quoted for when results begin to become apparent. Perseverance and commitment to the desired goal is paramount to achieving lasting positive changes.

Meditation is a uniquely personal experience, in much the same way as prayer can be. The inner world is richly diverse and fulfilling when we are given the opportunity for exploration. What we experience in our inner world will never be the same as is experienced by anyone else. Coming to know and trust the power of meditation takes time and consistent practice. No two meditations are alike. Each is an experience to be savored. With regular meditation there is resultant personal and spiritual growth. With continuing meditation you will become more attuned to the spiritual dimensions and meaning of life. It adds depth and comfort that is then extended and applied to the harshness of the physical reality, greatly enriching all life situations and experiences.

Introducing Meditation

If you have not yet enjoyed the wonderful inner experience of meditation, I suggest you begin simply. Explore several techniques. Try them out and then assess which feels the most comfortable for you. It is not necessary to sign up for expensive classes in order to find what you are seeking.

- Many yoga classes include a short period of relaxation at the end of the class. After a session of yoga breathing and stretching, this is a wonderful way of relaxing and introducing the meditative state into your awareness.

- Find a meditation class in your local neighborhood. Look for one that feels appropriate for your needs. Take time to explore what is being offered as there may be several techniques taught in different classes. Always allow intuition to be your guide in making a decision.

- A class situation offers the opportunity to explore, question, and share with others. This is a comfortable way of opening up to the meditation energies and to feel safe when delving into the inner consciousness in the initial stages.

- Prior to attending a class, it may be well worth learning more about the different meditation techniques. There are many books written on this subject and the Internet is another great source of information.

- There is an extensive range of meditation CDs and cassettes available for purchase. Often, a guided meditation assists in reducing the mind chatter, as listening to a soothing voice guiding the meditation becomes the focus and enables the body to go into a state of relaxation. I recommend purchasing at least one meditation CD for daily meditation practice. Allow yourself to become comfortable with focusing on breath and the guided meditation.

- Once you have become familiar and comfortable with guided meditations, you may choose to have only soft music playing in the background. This allows you to be fully in the meditative state without relying on a soothing voice to guide you through the process. With regular practice and focus, you will eventually reach a stage where you are able to meditate anywhere and without any guided meditations or music. The silence itself envelops and immerses you into the meditative state.

- Allot a regular time for meditation. For some people the morning is the best time, for others it is at the end of the day. Set aside regular time, and, if for some reason, there is an interruption to your schedule, reschedule the allotted meditation time.

Regular meditation practice is a must for anyone undergoing a process of self-healing. It facilitates, assists, and is integral to the healing process on all levels. By clearing the mind of accumulated chatter and clutter you are able to see more clearly exactly how you are creating your life, and with this awareness it becomes possible to change and create a life that is truly aligned to your heart's desire.

System Balancing (Refer to CD)

Sit comfortably in a chair with your back straight, legs uncrossed, and feet on the floor. Rest your arms gently on your lap. Concentrate on your breath. Breathe slowly and deeply. Feel your inhalation as it circulates throughout your body. With each exhalation, feel some of the stress you have been holding in your body releasing.

Now move your breath to a deeper level. Bring in white light with your inhalation and circulate it into each and every cell. Deeply inhale and hold your breath for the count of four. One. Two. Three. Four. On the exhalation release any stored emotions or stress sitting deep within the cellular level.

Visualize this process as a cycle. Inhale cleansing white light and exhale dark energy. Repeat this process a few times.

Continue breathing gently and slowly. As your body relaxes, your mind will also let go. Feel yourself release your inner dialogue. Leave all worries behind for a while. Allow your mind to reach a clear and calm space. In this relaxed state, your mind does not attach itself to distracting thoughts. Merely observe them and continue focusing on your relaxing and healing breath.

Now visualize a golden orb of spinning light above your head. This light is love and is your connection with the Divine Source. Focus your attention on this orb. Slowly bring it down through the top of your crown chakra along your body's mid-line. Feel the orb stop behind your third eye. Visualize it spinning strongly as it moves simultaneously toward both the back and front of your body and out to your energy field. The golden orb is an energy mass that spins continuously. Feel it clearing any blockages stored in the third eye chakra. Your third eye will continue spinning, radiating light energy, as blockages are released.

When you feel your third eye is clear and open, retract the golden orb and visualize it moving down to the throat chakra. Move the golden orb outward, to both the front and the back of your throat chakra. Feel the vibrant energy spinning outward in both directions. Feel your throat chakra being cleared and filled with light.

Continue bringing the spinning golden orb downward through the mid-line of your body. Stop at the heart center and feel the vibrant energy spinning outward in both directions. Feel your heart center being cleared and filled with light. Take a moment to feel the vibrant tingling within your body from your head down to your heart center as your chakras spin strongly. You are radiating light in all directions. This light appears to be white, but actually contains a universe of color.

From the heart center, move the golden orb of energy to your solar plexus. Again, direct the orb to the front and back of your solar plexus. You may have some difficulty with the lower chakras because the energy there is often deeply blocked. Imagine the energy moving outward to both front and back, like a growing ripple in a pool of water. As the ripples continue to grow, the energy blockage is eventually forced outward, clearing the chakra. When you feel you have done as much as possible, move to the sacral chakra, located just below the navel, and repeat the process. Feel the vibrant energy spinning outward in all directions. Feel your sacral chakra being cleared and filled with light.

Finally, move the spinning golden orb to your base chakra and repeat the process. Visualize the energy moving outward, clearing blockages, opening your base chakra and filling it with light.

From your base chakra, visualize the spinning golden orb moving down your legs, through your knees and calves, and into your feet. The energy spills out of your feet and becomes embedded, grounding and connecting you with Mother Earth as it continues to spin within all your chakras. Your whole energy field is filled with a mass of radiating light.

Concentrate on the energy of the orb below your feet, moving it upward and into your entire body again, infusing your being with surging, spinning light energy that radiates to all corners of your energy field. Your entire being and energy field are cleared and balanced, leaving you sustained and calm for the rest of your day.

CHAPTER THIRTEEN
Believing
and Creating

"One's own thought is one's world.
What a person thinks is what he becomes.
That is the eternal mystery."
—The Upanishads (800–600 BC)—

You believe what you know. What you come to know becomes your truth. Your view of what is true comes from your observation of the world and is greatly shaped by the beliefs and knowledge you have acquired. Quite some time ago, I encountered a simple truth that struck a significant chord with me. That saying is, "The world is what it is." This basically means that the world is what you believe it to be. Thus the perception you have of the world creates the life you lead. Ultimately, your perception shapes the reality and belief systems you hold.

The meaning you attach to life is determined by numerous factors including upbringing, background, and cultural values. Whatever you know continues to be adapted and modified according to life expectations and experiences. Usually, expectations determine your experiences, which in turn reinforce your belief systems. This is especially the case when you accept as truth your social conditioning, which is what most people do, without ever really probing deeply or questioning that this is the only or real truth.

It is important to be mindful of these concepts when you engage in the process of self-healing. Any journey of healing involves probing deeply into truths, perceptions, beliefs, attitudes, and values. It is only by questioning and discarding whatever is no longer relevant that a shift in perception can occur. When this takes place, the result is a release of old limitations and beliefs, which enables the engagement of meaningful and positive growth on the emotional, mental, and spiritual levels.

Prior to birth we are exposed to environmental factors and conditioning that impact early development and life perspective. A child that is wanted, loved, and nurtured while in the womb enters the world with that energy within and around it. A child that is unwanted and who is exposed to emotional, environmental, and other pollutants while in the womb carries that with him or her into the beginning of life. Whatever is experienced within the womb leaves an imprint, which is then generally reinforced through a multitude of life incidents and situations.

Infants and young children are highly sensitive to the energies of the environment into which they are born. They take on the values, attitudes, beliefs, and emotions that are common to their family and community group. There is no escaping it—you are hostage to the environment of your birth. It is from this environment that the richness and diversity of life are experienced. Whatever happens in the early formative years impacts upon personality, beliefs, perceptions, attitudes, and values. Humans are like large sponges, ready and willing to absorb all that is within the immediate vicinity. This occurs regardless of the individual's ability to discern between what is beneficial and what is detrimental to general well-being.

Young children, having greater sensitivity than adults, not only absorb the energies of their immediate family and surroundings but are able to sense, usually without understanding, a great deal of what happens outside their immediate world. These experiences become indelibly imprinted and are unique to the person experiencing them. In the space of a relatively short period of time, a myriad of emotions and perceptions are absorbed about the world and themselves. In addition, whatever has been brought into this lifetime is added to by whatever incidents are necessary for spiritual growth. By this I am referring to karma, past-life fears, experiences, and incidents that are to be continued into present life.

It is common for families to share specific and valued family traditions, whether they are favored celebrations or involve the passing down of precious mementos. Other family traditions also exist that are not necessarily verbally acknowledged. In most instances, there is not even the awareness that a tradition is being perpetuated. These are, in particular, the traditions that relate to health and well-being. In recent years there has been more public acknowledgment of the role that family beliefs around health can have in influencing an individual's future health status. In addition, there are powerful subtle traditions, attitudes, behaviors, and values that are maintained from generation to generation. Fears, insecurities, anger, and other intense emotional and behavioral responses and patterns are impressed unconsciously by the adult and strongly internalized by the young impressionable child. This process of internalization in unavoidable and is experienced by everyone.

As you embark upon this wonderful journey called life, you attract further incidents and experiences that solidify earlier internalized experiences and insights about life and its meaning. These reinforce your beliefs and perceptions. Situations and incidents arise that verify earlier observations, so it is relatively easy to draw clear conclusions about life. The emotional component is an integral part of this process. Consequently, a buildup of incidents, issues, and perceptions accumulates that eventually results in strongly held feelings about the nature and structure of reality.

In addition to family values, those promulgated by the wider society impinge greatly on your consciousness. Scant reference has been made so far to the role of media, advertising, and the influence of large multinational corporations in shaping the lives of people. Their influence cannot be underestimated nor readily overcome. Their sway has become insidious on practically every level.

Without doubt, advertising and consumerism shape general societal values and beliefs. If you were to seek corroboration of this claim, a visit to any city or town in the United States would attest to this statement. Most communities boast the same mega-stores promoting their particular wares and countless identical fast-food outlets that promote a particular way of eating. As a society, and individually, we have become conditioned to accept a certain standard and way of living, irrespective of what its long-term and lasting impact is.

For example, drinking coffee and sodas, eating danishes and donuts are considered the norm, and this is despite the fact that people will often say, as they are indulging in these foods, that these foods are unhealthy and should be avoided. The practice continues because certain goods and foods are mass-produced, are readily available, and, most importantly, are culturally encouraged. Where does this cultural acceptance stem from? It is not necessary to be another Sherlock Holmes or Einstein to see the obvious link in advertising with consumer spending and lifestyles.

Have you ever questioned what is really happening to our basic lifestyle and common values? Do you question who or what is gaining from these gradual changes that are being force-fed on the general population? Do you ever question why the usual response from the population is meek acceptance? Even when there is momentary concern, or outrage, expressed about consumerism trends, advertising influences, and long-term implications, it does not last long and the majority of people continue as before without making significant changes in lifestyle and purchasing habits. The reality is that the market will always provide whatever the consumer considers acceptable.

It is not only consumer habits that are driven by advertising and profit-driven companies. The influence of large corporations shapes the general public's beliefs and perception of issues, incidents, and products through the subtle means used by the media to carry a story. There are currently many stories being reported via the media that reinforce the belief that the world is not a safe place. Fear, anxiety, and mistrust are generated within a large population that is continually exposed to, and adopts, a diet of manufactured consensus. This influence and its implications for societal values are extensive and has been explored elsewhere.[23]

When there is a combination of beliefs that have been accepted as truths, due to consistent media coverage and expression, along with underlying anxiety and fear, then is it any wonder that a myriad of twentieth-century ill health conditions are proliferating? The individual, after exposure to innumerable emotions and beliefs from early years, is already endeavoring to make some sense of what appears to be a chaotic world. The added fears and insecurities from advertising and media bombardment can only reinforce limiting beliefs about the self.

As explained in chapter 5, everything initially impacts the energy field prior to registering and becoming established on the physical level. The emotional, mental, and spiritual levels register a response to whatever happens. This response is felt within the energy field and then stored within the complex and sensitive energy grid. The energy field is basically a storehouse of information, containing the energy of all thoughts, emotions, issues, and beliefs.

As an example, a young child may strongly sense fear in a parent and that fear then registers in his or her energy field. Life situations and issues will continue to induce other fear reactions, which in turn will be stored within the energy field. Eventually, when confronted by a situation that may require strength and quick problem solving skills,

---

23. For further information, see: Noam Chomsky and Edward S. Herman, *Manufacturing Consent*, Pantheon Press, 1998; and Charles Derber, *Corporation Nation: How Corporations Are Taking Over Our Lives—And What We Can Do About It*, St. Martin's Press, 2000.

that individual will instinctively react fearfully and may even be paralyzed by fear as it permeates the body. The accumulation of fear from a lifetime of fear-based reactions creates a predominance of that energy within the energy field. Fear then underpins that individual's response to practically every life situation. The example of fear is used because it is imbued within many beliefs and perceptions held by the average person. For this reason, a later chapter has been devoted to exploring the insidiousness of fear.

Many beliefs originate in the formative years, and these are created for survival purposes. They were appropriate at that time and were adopted to ensure continued existence in the best possible manner. Once into adulthood, there is generally no further need for a great number of those beliefs. They are no longer essential to survival because adults are able to deal with life issues in a more appropriate manner. With that awareness, it then becomes easy to make the choice to let go of limiting beliefs and old conditioning.

It has been my practice to become a witness to my own emotions and beliefs. This occurs by observing whatever emotions and reactions are being experienced. Depending on the situation and reaction, a number of core questions are then asked. These questions can apply to practically any situation.

- Why do I believe this?
- What is the belief underlying this emotion or reaction?
- Is there any truth to the belief?
- What is the truth?
- Where does this belief originate?
- Does this belief serve me well now?
- If not, what is the appropriate belief (and behavior) to replace it with?

You will find, when adopting this approach to understanding the beliefs you hold, that there is not necessarily any immediate diminishing of emotion or reaction. There is, instead, greater awareness and insight as your intuitive knowing releases buried memories of earlier incidents and issues. These will rise to the surface of your consciousness with clarity. From this, greater understanding is reached, and eventually over time there is a considerable reduction in unwarranted emotional reactions and outbursts.

Becoming the observer of your emotions is an empowering practice. Whenever there is an emotional response to a situation, allow yourself the opportunity to observe what is happening. Take note of the immediate thoughts that come to mind as to the real cause of the reaction. Sometimes it may be necessary to ask yourself several questions about the origin and reason for such an emotional response. Slowly and with persistence, a picture of the real issues, beliefs, or fears underlying the emotional response will emerge.

The more being an observer is practiced, the easier it becomes to recognize almost instantly not only the origin of the emotion but also often the extremity of any intense reaction. In most instances the response is usually all out of proportion to the trigger that brought it to consciousness.

Gentle Awareness Technique

The use of visualization to create awareness of underlying beliefs that cause negative emotions or reactions is a powerful tool. This is a different process to becoming a witness or observer to a response you experience. Being an observer relies more on analysis and reasoning. The visualization allows you to engage the emotions and determine where the underlying belief originated. This visualization will assist you to become aware of the beliefs you hold that no longer serve you well. The next chapter contains exercises and strategies to release and clear outmoded beliefs.

1. Find a restful position. Focus on slow and calm breathing, allowing your whole body to totally relax.

2. Focus your mind on an emotion or reaction that you wish to change. Visualize when it last occurred. Calmly note your responses.

3. Now focus your mind back to a previous time when you experienced the same emotion or reaction. Observe the situation and intuitively

feel whether there was a similar trigger that provoked the reaction.

4. Continue this process of focusing the mind backward to earlier times and the situations that provoked a similar response. In each situation, calmly feel your emotional response. You are not reliving the experience, merely acknowledging the emotion.

5. Begin to visualize the connection between each situation and your emotional response. You will find a common thread, which will ultimately highlight how you acquired a certain belief. This process will also demonstrate how this particular belief has been reinforced throughout many life experiences.

6. Once you have gained insight into the origins of the particular belief you have explored, you will probably have an "ah ha" moment when you experience great knowing and possibly even some emotional pain. Do not remain in that state. Remind yourself that you are no longer in a place of pain—you are now in a place of healing. That gentle reminder will assist you back into a space of calmness.

7. Allow yourself several deep, relaxing breaths in which you focus only on your breathing. Then slowly come out of the visualization.

Whenever you experience an emotional response that you feel is inappropriate or detrimental to your well-being, repeat this process. You will find there will invariably be an underlying belief responsible. Use this process to empower yourself. With the insight and understanding gained, you will find that irrational and unwarranted emotional responses will diminish.

CHAPTER FOURTEEN
Releasing Limitations

"There is tranquility in ignorance,
but servitude is its partner."
—George Duisman—

In my field of work, a considerable percentage of my clients seek healing for old and deep-seated emotional wounds. They search for understanding and resolution of long-held pain, relationship dysfunction, and other related emotional and mental conditions. There are a number of limiting beliefs common to clients due to conditioning, life experiences, and the internalization process. My suspicion is that some or all of these beliefs would most probably be shared, to some degree, by a majority of the population. It should be noted that these limiting beliefs are not necessarily readily evident to the individual who holds them. They tend to be trapped in the subconscious, from which they regularly appear in many disguises in order to sabotage higher ideals and aspirations.

These beliefs are limiting because they limit our true potential. They can prevent us from experiencing life to its fullest. Carried to the extreme, one or several limiting beliefs can contribute to ill health. A belief is insubstantial. It is based upon perception. Nothing more or less. Nevertheless, beliefs are energy, and as energy they will manifest in the form we give them. As energy, they are also stored in the complex energy grid, though they can be released.

You will clearly see from the following list of limiting beliefs that you can choose to change any that are affecting your life. Each description also contains strategies for releasing the beliefs. When you begin working in the manner suggested, you are working with energy. You are using energy to move energy!

Lack of Self-Worth

Lack of self-worth is a common limiting belief. The perception is that you are not good enough, not worthy enough, not pretty enough, not interesting enough, lack talent, skill, and intellect, and so on. The focus is on whatever is perceived to be lacking. Simple messages received throughout earlier years and reinforced by life experiences convincingly cement this belief. No matter what the perceived lack, ultimately this belief has the potential to teach you to value the self.

In our culture it is easy to speak without thinking about the possible consequences of whatever is expressed. This is due largely to the fact that it is socially desirable to be both expressive and articulate. The art of heeding the thoughts before they are expressed is not taught. Nor is the art of listening and reflection valued and taught. At thirteen years of age, an acquaintance was told by his art teacher that he could not draw. The words were internalized and the only drawing attempts even contemplated after that was an occasional doodle on a notepad. It was not until this acquaintance was much older that he enrolled in a recreation class where he learned to draw using the right side of the brain. It was then that the extent of the damage created by his teacher's words became evident. During the class his drawing abilities blossomed rapidly, and the realization set in that a simple statement all those years ago had convinced him he lacked all artistic talent, thus depriving him of many wonderful opportunities.

At times the message given is that you are stupid, other times you may be compared unfavorably with siblings or classmates, and sometimes you may compare yourself as inferior to other people's talents, personalities and appearances. All these lead to low self-esteem, which in most instances is masked from the world around you. Eventually the low self-esteem will undermine your performance at critical instances in your life. Whenever you experience feelings of inadequacy, the inherent belief is lack of self-worth.

Lack of self-worth affects both the mental and emotional levels. Your mind toys with notions of unworthiness. Self-talk becomes negative and denigrating and, if continued incessantly, can ultimately lead to feelings of depression. On the emotional level, lack of self-worth is expressed as fear, negativity, judgment, criticism, hatred, envy, defensiveness, and even arrogance and overconfidence. The energy field becomes weighed down with the energy of these negative thoughts and emotions, especially when they are accumulated over a lifetime!

At all times both the physical body and the energy field strive to be in balance. When the energy field is filled with negativity, it eventually affects the physical body in some manner. This is the body's way of telling us that some aspect of our lives is out of balance and needs to be addressed and healed.

Suggested Strategies

1. Complete the visualization exercise outlined in the previous chapter. This will assist you to gain insight about incidents that have triggered a lack of self-worth.

2. Quietly acknowledge that you coped as best as you could at that time. Then affirm you are now an adult and that it is time to let go of beliefs that served you well when you were younger and are no longer appropriate.

3. Make a declaration of release. This will facilitate the release of the stuck energy. You may choose your own meaningful statement or use this statement: "I release with love all emotions and thoughts that have contributed to my lack of self-worth. I release them from all times, all dimensions, and all planes. I replace them with the energy of unconditional love, and I know that the universe provides abundance in all things."

4. Old habits have a way of resurfacing, and you have the power to change old patterns. Whenever the thought intrudes that you are not good enough, lack talent, and so on, then affirm aloud the exact opposite. Affirm that you are beautiful, that you are deserving, and so on.

5. Write a list of all your special skills and talents. Write another list of your delightful qualities. Write yet another list describing how other people see you. You have more beautiful attributes than you realize. Listing them is very revealing. If you have an awareness of some negative qualities that you wish to change, write them as a positive statement and describe how you will achieve this intended change. Refer to these lists as often as you choose. Use them in affirming ways in everyday life situations. Continual reinforcement of your worth will pay dividends.

Self-Hatred

Feelings of self-hatred or dislike are other limiting beliefs. A young woman, holding a lot of inner tension and anger, came as a client. Her family and work life appeared to be satisfying and harmonious. The reason for her inner tension was revealed when she blurted out, "I hate myself." This young woman was incredibly slim, highly personable, intelligent, and extremely attractive but could not see that in herself. She held the perception that she was ugly. This perception was based on incidents that had occurred in her younger years.

Self-dislike or self-hatred is a widespread belief held by a large proportion of the population. Learning to like and even to love yourself is anathema to societal conditioning. It is far easier to focus your love exclusively on immediate family and friends than it is to acknowledge that you love and value yourself.

When the energy of self-hatred is present in an individual, that energy emanates outwardly and will in its own way attract people of a similar inclination. In personal and intimate relationships this is not the most desirable recipe for a successful and lasting union. It is similar with friendships, as eventually self-hatred will reveal itself in emotional outbursts that create a schism in communication and can then lead to a lack of trust. Self-hatred is a destructive force. It is soul destroying. Negative messages from thoughts and emotions are sent throughout the physical body and the energy field and impede the flow of love, thereby creating disharmony and pain. The physical body and the energy field are like a hothouse plant. Nourishment (love) is needed for survival, growth, and well-being. Sadly, we live in a world where hatred is commonly expressed. It is accepted as normal to hate or dislike. These emotions involve judgment and criticism.

Imagine a delicious meal that is being served to you. The person who has prepared it is filled with self-hatred and is holding onto a lot of anger and resentment. Will you detect this energy in the meal? If you are sensitive to energies and vibes, the food will taste like ash, and most likely you will not be inclined to eat a great deal. If, however, the person preparing the meal cooks with love, then the food is imbued with that energy, and your response to the meal will be highly favorable. Whatever you feel and think is held within your energy field and is easily felt and identified by other people.

Suggested Strategies

1. Complete the visualization exercise outlined in the previous chapter. This will assist to you gain insight to the incidents that have triggered the feeling of self-hatred.

2. Acknowledge that you coped as best as you could at that time. Then affirm you are now an adult and that it is time to let go of beliefs that served you well when you were younger.

3. Declare a statement of release. This will facilitate healing. You may choose your own meaningful statement or use this statement: "I release with love all emotions and thoughts that have contributed to my self-hatred. I release them from all times, all dimensions, and all planes. I replace them with unconditional love and know that I am a vessel for love in all my endeavors and intentions."

4. Use affirmations of self-love at every possible opportunity. Think and speak only positively about yourself. When negative thoughts intrude, observe where they come from and then lovingly replace them with a positive and nourishing affirmation.

5. When other people speak disparagingly to you or about you, be assertive about your worth. It is important that you honor the feelings of self-love and acceptance.

6. Align your behaviors with the energy of self-love. Frequently ask, "Does this action serve my highest good?" If not, then discontinue that behavior.

7. Support yourself through this process by continually assessing what is nourishing and self-loving. Whenever possible, reinforce your new way of viewing yourself with rewards. The use of rewards is a reminder that you are in a state of self-love and acceptance and not in a state of deprivation. You may choose to have a bodywork session, treat yourself to a movie, or do something else that enhances the feeling of self-love.

Victimhood

The limiting belief of victimhood is displayed in people of varying backgrounds. Believing that any misfortune suffered is the result of life circumstances, genes, past behaviors, family, and others' moods places you in a position where you are absolved from taking responsibility for whatever transpires in your life. Victimhood creates disempowerment in all life situations. Victimhood is a gradual process. Over time you come to expect others to rectify life issues and problems.

A woman I met was unhappy with her life. She was in an abusive relationship and had learned to modify her behavior so she wouldn't aggravate her husband. She accepted the blame whenever he was irritated and devoted effort to ensuring his needs were met. In conversation she admitted she was unwilling to change anything. The security of marriage was more important than creating change to find happiness. Clients often express similar attitudes. Sometimes parents feel they are hostage to their children's demands, yet feel their children's happiness is a priority and are so unwilling to set boundaries for acceptable behavior. Others accuse their parents, upbringing, employer, society, and so on for a whole range of conditions and situations.

Energetically, whenever you engage in victimhood, you are actually manifesting emotions of anger, resentment, blame, criticism, and judgment. Victimhood occurs on the emotional level, though the consequences will likely affect the mental and spiritual levels. If the victimhood behaviors persist throughout life, the resultant emotions fester deeply and may eventually manifest as physical illness. Every time victimhood behavior takes place, the emotions register within the energy field and place stress on the energy grid itself. Simultaneously, your sense of self is diminished. From an energy perspective, your vitality is reduced. Expending energy in negative emotions robs the energy field of the vitality that is needed for healthy functioning.

When you stop blaming others and begin to seriously question your actions and beliefs, you are able to observe realistically what is actually happening and from that an opportunity for change and growth in interpersonal relationships is created.

Suggested Strategies

1. Complete the visualization exercise outlined in the previous chapter. This will assist you to gain insight to the reasons why you feel as though other people or other circumstances are responsible for whatever has happened in your life.

2. Become an observer to your behavior around people. Do you compromise your feelings? Do you continually say "sorry" even when you are not responsible? Do you feel powerless with certain people or situations? Through assessing your interpersonal interactions, you will soon be able to identify those that diminish you in some way.

3. As the observer, you will begin to discern certain patterns. It may be that you continually feel responsible for ensuring everyone's enjoyment or happiness while denying your needs. Or you may feel angry with certain people or circumstances that have occurred in your life and continually cast the blame elsewhere. Observe the patterns of your responses and beliefs. It may be worth keeping a log of incidents and your emotions.

4. Determine which responses and behaviors no longer feel appropriate and then make the changes accordingly. Whatever changes you implement should always be positive and affirming.

5. Check your emotional responses. When you find anger, judgment, and criticism toward other people or situations, acknowledge that emotion as yours, and no one else's. Take responsibility for owning the emotion. Then deal with it. There are ample exercises and suggestions included in this book to assist you. Once you have done this, the pattern of victimhood will diminish.

External Validation

It is easy to hold the belief that other people know what is best for you. This is what is subconsciously taught from the time you are young and dependent on adults to make decisions regarding your welfare. Looking to other people to validate decisions or opinions tends to continue into adulthood and is commonplace within most social contexts. The desire to be accepted by others seems to be inherently powerful in all people. Yet, in seeking external validation it is easy to overlook or deny what is internally true for you.

When you continually strive for external validation, it is easy to lose sight of your inner strength and therefore deplete your self-confidence. Seeking external validation results in disempowerment. Seeking approval and corroboration for your decisions and behavior inevitably results in further chaos and confusion in life. No one else knows exactly what is most appropriate for you. Someone else can only say what he or she thinks is best. That judgment is based on their experiences and perceptions, which are not necessarily in harmony with your highest good.

You are a spirit being having a human experience and are here to learn who you really are and what your purpose is. The only way to truly begin to gain this insight is to listen to your inner voice. Doing this involves following your inner voice or intuition that wells up instinctively from time to time. Listening to this voice is the first step. Learning to heed it is the next step. When doing this there will be many changes in life circumstances that will lead to gradual improvement.

Seeking external validation robs your autonomy, depletes your power, and weakens you energetically. The person continually seeking validation actually has some degree of low self-worth, which was covered at the beginning of the chapter. The opposite occurs when you possess genuine self-confidence, which is empowering and generates feelings of strength and wellness.

Suggested Strategies

1. Complete the visualization exercise outlined the in previous chapter. This will assist you to gain insight to the incidents that have triggered the need for external validation.

2. Acknowledge that you coped as best as you could at that time and that you have learned valuable lessons from the experiences.

Then affirm that you are now an adult and that it is time to let go of beliefs that no longer serve you.

3. Make a statement of release to facilitate healing. You may choose your own meaningful statement or state the following: "I release with love all beliefs, emotions, and thoughts that have created my need for external validation. I release them from all times, all dimensions, and all planes. I replace them with unconditional love and know that I am confident and able to make decisions for my highest good in all situations. I now allow myself to be guided by my inner voice and intuitive knowing."

4. Use affirmations to support your growing self-confidence.

5. Learn to be discerning. When other people express their opinions about you, thank them for their consideration. Know that they have expressed their opinion. They own the opinion—you are responsible only for how you choose to feel and act.

6. Speak your truth, even when it is contrary to what is expressed by other people. If you have difficulty with this initially, rehearse your lines beforehand. Practice in front of a mirror or with a trusted friend.

7. Learn to listen to and heed your inner voice. It is always available and it is a matter of becoming familiar with the advice and guidance dispensed. The more you respond to your inner voice, or intuition, the greater your confidence will become.

Other People's Emotions

Taking responsibility and self-blame for other people's emotions of anger, frustration, disappointment, irritation, and so on is another limiting belief. This is an instinctive response and is most likely linked to conditioning from earlier years. Young children are highly sensitive to intense adult emotions. When listening to adults reflecting on their childhood years, it is common to hear them express the responsibility they felt around their parents' anger or abusive behavior.

You do not make other people unhappy, irritated, disappointed, or angry. You have not done something wrong if they choose to behave in a specific negative way. This is an important point. You choose your emotions, though in most instances they appear to occur reflexively, unconsciously, and instinctively. No one else makes you feel a certain way. It is a common misperception that someone may make you angry, sad, or happy. Emotions come from thoughts. In most instances you feel anger, sadness, and so on because of a subconscious belief or conditioning that is held.

A friend began exhibiting intense anger, mostly at inappropriate times. It seemed that very little was needed to stimulate an angry outburst. She eventually chose to fathom a reason for the intense and sudden rages. She realized that, as a child, she had learned to always be on her best behavior. Her father, in particular, made it absolutely clear that life had to be lived according to his rules. Many childhood incidents arose where she had a choice of being compliant or of speaking her truth. It did not take long to understand the consequences of being headstrong, so the decision to be meek and compliant was the easier of the two options. She internalized her father's deep anger, believing she was responsible for his outbursts. Consequently, she learned to suppress anger, and by the time she was in her forties, the stored anger began erupting. Once that awareness registered, she was able to release the anger in an appropriate and safe manner.

Believing you are responsible for someone else's emotions diminishes your energy field. This is another form of victimhood and disempowers you from living your truth. Your energy field thrives on positive energy. Any discordant energy has the opposite effect. On an emotional level, this limiting belief can have a debilitating effect on self-esteem and worth. When strong emotions are suppressed, they remain within the energy field and, if not healed, will eventually manifest in some form of illness.

Suggested Strategies

1. Complete the visualization exercise outlined in the previous chapter. This will assist you to gain insight to the incidents

and situations that have resulted in your feeling responsible for someone else's emotions and moods.

2. Acknowledge that you coped as best as you could at that time and that you have learned valuable lessons from the experiences. Then affirm that you are now an adult and that it is time to let go of beliefs that no longer serve you.

3. Make a statement of release to facilitate healing. You may choose your own meaningful statement or state the following: "I release with love all beliefs, emotions, and thoughts that have created my belief that I am responsible for the emotions and moods of other people. I release them from all times, all dimensions, and all planes. I replace them with unconditional love and I know that I am responsible only for my beliefs, emotions, thoughts, and actions."

4. Whenever you find yourself feeling some degree of responsibility for emotions and moods exhibited by another person, affirm that you are responsible for only your emotions, thoughts, beliefs, behaviors, and so on.

5. If it is appropriate, state your non-responsibility to the person involved. This is relevant where the person indicates that you are the reason for their emotion, mood, or behavior. In most instances it is likely that the person is unaware of what you are experiencing.

Self-Denial

A powerful limiting belief is that your needs and desires are not of paramount importance. It is easy to subjugate your needs and wishes to those of others, especially the needs of family and close community. Prioritizing self-care and desires can be perceived as being self-centered, thoughtless of others, and negligent of your responsibilities. There is no denying that the ability to live cooperatively and supportively is a wonderful human trait. Caring for others is commendable and highly desirable within all societies. This is why the trait of giving service to others is encouraged from an early age. It is when this trait is carried to an extreme and your particular needs and desires are neglected that there is a resultant imbalance in some area of your life. In many instances service becomes an onerous duty. When this is the case, there is every chance of deep-seated resentment festering.

Many adults reach a point in their life when they question the meaning of life. Having devoted many years to the care and demands of their family, there is a realization that there is a lack of purpose. Or they may have lost sight of a long-cherished dream. In such situations it is acceptable to focus on the self for a while and to ensure the needs and aspirations of the inner self are fulfilled. When the inner self becomes filled with purpose and life has real meaning, then they are in a balanced emotional state and better able to serve and honor others.

You have a specific purpose or path in this life. Living your life according to the expectations and demands of others will not assist you to achieve this. It is only when there is awareness of your purpose and you align your life accordingly that you are able to achieve real meaning, passion, and joy in all aspects of life. When experiencing this state, it becomes easy to have more compassion, understanding, and acceptance of others and their unique journey. You come to value their special spirit without denigrating or devaluing yours in any way.

When giving priority to the needs of others while neglecting your own, you are actually giving a message that you are not important! This, yet again, is another aspect of the limiting belief around lack of self-worth. This message is felt within your energy field as your energy is continually directed outward toward supplying the needs of other people. You are literally giving your energy away in order to sustain their needs or desires, thereby depleting your own reservoir. In order to survive, your energy field requires ongoing sustenance, much like your physical body. Without this there will be a weakening of the energy grid structures. In time, as mentioned previously, there is the likelihood of deep resentment and anger surfacing, and this will manifest in some manner. In such situations it is essential to focus on healing the cause of the ill health as well as the form in which it has manifested.

Suggested Strategies

1. Complete the visualization exercise outlined in the previous chapter. This will assist you to gain insight to the incidents and situations that have resulted in the denial or suppression of your needs.

2. Acknowledge that you coped as best as you could at that time and that you have learned valuable lessons from the experiences. Then affirm that you are now an adult and that it is time to let go of beliefs that no longer serve you.

3. Make a statement of release to facilitate healing. You may choose your own meaningful statement or state the following: "I release with love all beliefs, emotions, and thoughts that have created my belief that the needs and desires of other people are my responsibility. I release this belief from all times, all dimensions, and all planes. I replace this belief with unconditional love and take responsibility for fulfilling my life purpose."

4. In your daily routine, create time for yourself. Allot time for activities that are important to your self-growth and ensure that this time is not violated by the demands of others.

5. Learn to express your needs to people who are important in your life. Positive and assertive sharing is empowering. When you value your needs, you will find that people will respect and value them as well.

Conditioned behaviors and responses weaken when you reach understanding and acceptance of the origins of your beliefs. When this occurs, a state of empowerment results. It becomes possible to create a new set of beliefs that are more aligned with your current situation, your life purpose, and a reality that is based in the essence of harmony and truth.

Overcoming a limiting belief requires both commitment and time. However, the effort is well worth it. When such a belief is released, you are able to expand and explore life no longer hindered by conditioned responses and behaviors. The strategies for dealing with each limiting belief are to be used as a guide only. This is your journey of exploration and healing. Allow yourself to be guided by your inner voice. When you feel an urge or desire to explore in ways other than those suggested, by all means follow that inner guidance. The more that limiting beliefs are released, the more energized you will feel. Gradually you will feel strengthened within. This will be a positive rather than depleted feeling, and it is an indication that your energy field is receiving sustenance through your constructive endeavors.

Healing Harmony (Refer to CD)

Find a quiet place where you are comfortable sitting, standing, or lying. Close your eyes and let a feeling of deep relaxation move through your eyes and into the muscles in your face. Feel tension leaving your head from your neck and shoulders. Consciously bring your awareness to any tension you hold within your body and begin to release it by inhaling deeply. As you exhale, feel all of your muscles deeply relax. Continue releasing tension until your whole body is completely calm and relaxed.

Continue breathing gently and deeply. Be aware of the energy within and around you as you remain in a relaxed state. Your mind should be as calm and clear as your body. If not, focus your intention again on your breath, inhaling and exhaling until you are able to put your thoughts to rest.

While you are breathing, be aware of what is happening within your body, then consciously identify an area of pain you would like to heal, whether it is an instance of physical or emotional pain. Bring your awareness to this specific pain. Leave all other thoughts behind and calmly observe the emotions you hold around the pain; do not feel the emotions. In your totally relaxed state, you are able to observe your pain without feeling it directly.

Now that you have an awareness of the pain you wish to heal, find where it is located in your body. If it is a physical condition, you may feel it in more than one area. If it is emotional, it may sit in any of the lower three chakras, or even in your heart center.

When you have located the area where the pain resides, bring your attention to your energy field. Feel the energies within and around you flowing freely. Sense the interconnectedness between your physical body and your energy field. You expand your consciousness by becoming more aware of your physical, mental, emotional, and energetic bodies.

With your consciousness expanded, can you feel if the pain you have isolated exists within your energy field? Visualize the pain encapsulated within a ball in front of you, about twelve inches from your heart center. Clearly identify where your emotion around this pain sits within your energy field. Know that it has revealed itself because it is ready to be released.

Bring your awareness to your heart center, which is slightly to the right of your physical heart. The energy in your heart center is spinning strongly. Visualize your heart center opening as you begin to feel the energy moving outward in a vortex. Feel the love in your heart center spilling out, like a soft, pink fountain, gradually filling your entire energy field.

Now harness this pink energy flow and direct it to the pain you have identified. Totally surround the pain with pink light. Wrap it in pink as you would wrap a package, then feel the force of the energy flow as it continues surging outward, carrying your pain away. Feel the sensation of pain leaving your body and your energy field. You may see what is happening in your energy grid during this process. Feel the pulling sensation as the release occurs, knowing that your pain has been released to a higher power. Quietly give thanks for its release.

As this is happening, visualize the pink light washing away any other unneeded negativity and emotions. Be aware of the changes occurring in your energy field. As you feel the release, continue focusing on your breathing, and then feel the lightness in the area where you released the pain. Visualize golden light streaming into your body and overflowing from this space. See your energy grid restored to a state of balance. You feel a deep inner quiet and calm. Remain there for as long as you choose.

The issue of fear and its related influence and impact on conditioning and belief systems has not been mentioned so far. Fear underlies countless aspects of daily life. It permeates many of the messages that are received constantly from all directions. It shapes and creates individual and shared reality. Because of its insidiousness and pervasiveness, fear is a topic that deserves deeper analysis and discussion and will be explored in a later chapter.

CHAPTER FIFTEEN

As You Think, So It Is

"We are what we think.
With our thoughts, we make the world."
—*Buddha*—

How you feel about yourself and your life will provide some important clues as to how you apply energy to everyday life. What is the first feeling you generally experience upon waking up? What sort of mood do you usually take to bed with you? Your honest response to these questions will provide you with clues about the energy you hold within your energy field. It is most likely that you experience a mix of emotions, some negative and some positive. Or you may even carry a dominance of one or the other.

Your feelings will provide an indication as to what is really happening in your life. Before proceeding any further, spend a minute or so reflecting on your immediate responses to the two questions. Then check whether your feelings and perceptions now are similar to what they were a month ago, twelve months ago, and even further back in your life. Have they changed in any way? If they have changed, what do you believe is the reason for this? Finally, what are the factors that have created the specific feelings you hold about life?

As you continue reading this and the following chapter, please keep in mind your responses to the above questions and your feelings about life in general. By doing this, you will be in a position to gain greater understanding of the following information and its relevance to your life. It is highly likely that you may already know a great deal of what is shared in my writing. So many times, when working with people, I hear them say, "I know," when my intuitive sense is that certain changes in lifestyle would be beneficial to their health and well-being. Be aware that knowing something is not necessarily the same thing as living it. The difference is enormous!

Society places a high value on knowing data, facts, and truths—especially when that knowledge is derived from book learning and scientific research. This form of knowing is, again, external to the self. It is actually what has been learned and is not true inner knowing, which is entirely different. It is easy enough to quote verbatim the wisdom of great sages and masters and to reel off data to substantiate your position or perspective on some aspect of life. Quoting what you have read and learned does not necessarily indicate that you truly know something.

When you really know something, it is because you have experienced it and understand the depth contained within the acquired knowledge.

Recently, someone close to me was astounded by a profound realization he had just experienced. His search for meaning spanned more than twenty years of seeking and studying. He could quote masters and teachings with great proficiency. However, the difference between learning universal truths and wisdom and actually knowing how to fully integrate them into daily living had eluded him. One day the realization struck that there is a significant difference between learning something, being able to discuss it knowledgeably, and actually living it as an inner knowing. Needless to say, his immediate concern then became how to best incorporate his knowing into living it as his truth.

What is shared in this and the following two chapters relates to your ability to create the life you richly deserve. I trust you will take the time to truly digest the information on reality creation. Absorb its meaning fully and then assess its implications for your life choices. The basic time-proven techniques described for creating a positive, healthy, and balanced life are well worth adopting. A commitment to making some degree of change is essential for success.

If, for some reason, there are areas in your life you are dissatisfied with, it is your responsibility to make appropriate changes in order to create improvement. It is all too easy to talk volubly about existing problems, but that does not ensure the necessary changes are implemented. Unfortunately it is often easier to blame other people or circumstances than it is to actively rectify the problems. Living with pain and discomfort can actually be more comfortable for some people than implementing meaningful change. The thought of making changes can be disconcerting and fearful. However, making small meaningful changes, even one at a time, can make a considerable difference to your quality of life.

So I encourage you to take the plunge. Assess where change would be beneficial to your health and well-being. Make a commitment to implement relevant changes in your daily life. Set achievable goals for yourself and then begin the process of creating a new and exciting reality that is more aligned with your higher aspirations and values.

Creating Reality

It is essential to be continually mindful of the fact that everything is energy. Every word, emotion, thought, and action carries energy. Those random and often confused thoughts that seemingly come from nowhere create your verbal and emotional expressions and also manifest as actions. They are somewhat like the paint that is splashed upon the canvas to create a picture. When the paint is splashed randomly, the result is likely to end up looking chaotic and disorganized, and the canvas is then open to multiple interpretations. Yet when there is forethought and clarity around the end result, the paint is applied more methodically and creatively. When this is the case, the final result is aesthetically pleasing, and you know intuitively what the artist intended.

The majority of people will deny they have created the life they're leading. In many instances they will attribute their problems to external factors. They protest that they would never create their lack of financial security, would not wish for the ill health they're experiencing, could not have created the family strife and misfortune that has beset them, and so on. On the conscious level of intent, that may very well be true. If there is a choice between financial security and financial insecurity, the preferred choice is obvious. The same applies for good health and ill health or any other situation where there is an element of duality. In reality, people generally desire happiness, love, abundance, peace, and all the wonderfully positive aspects of life. It is not as if there is a conscious and deliberate decision to create hardship. Hardship and pain happen because generally people have become unaware of the consequences of language usage.

Language Creates Reality

It is common to lose sight of the amazing power generated from the language we normally use. As energy, your thoughts, emotions, and words will do whatever it is that you create with them. Language can be used for positive or negative intent. Be aware that there is a universal law involved in this process. Whatever you give you also receive;

whatever you give to others will return to you in some form. Even the most innocuous thought that flits across your mind is energy and has a powerful influence. If nothing else, this means that it is all the more important to engage in regular meditation practice as this helps clear the mind of all the stored clutter that constantly creates meaningless and contradictory chatter!

Common expressions are used regularly in conversation without conscious awareness, as is demonstrated in the following instance. A friend of mine knew a woman who had the habit of beginning many of her sentences with the phrase "I can't stand . . ." This phrase may have been used to indicate a discomfort with the heat or maybe intolerance to certain foods, people, or behaviors. The underlying intent is irrelevant, but the words "I can't stand" over a period of time were absorbed initially into her energy field and finally into her body. Eventually she fell and broke both ankles so she literally could not stand!

Other examples I hear people use to describe feelings or situations include: "There's not enough time," "I am asthmatic/diabetic" (or some other condition), "It's so hard/difficult," "There's never enough money," "The world's not safe," "I'm too busy," and so on. Whatever you think or say happens. So, if you constantly say, "It's so hard," then that is most definitely what life becomes. You literally create your perception of life and reality from words and thoughts used randomly and unthinkingly.

A number of years ago when I was guided to learn Reiki, the teacher asked participants to share something about themselves with the rest of the group. The vast majority of people shared stories of ill health and made statements such as, "I am a diabetic," "I have asthma," and "My heart is weak." In every instance the teacher immediately asked them to rephrase their statement to indicate that their condition was a thing of the past. Instead of "I am a diabetic," they were told to say "I was a diabetic" or whatever their condition may have been.

By continually reiterating that you have a specific medical condition, learning impediment, or physical limitation, you are reinforcing that very perception within every level. The belief travels from the conscious to the subconscious mind and then settles comfortably into the energy field, which in turn then reaffirms the stated condition by its very responses and behaviors within the body.

This point is particularly relevant for anyone seeking to heal a specific health condition. Changing the language (and belief) around the condition is vitally important to the healing process. There are countless stories of people who have overcome incredible odds to make an amazing recovery, regardless of medical prognosis. Inherent in most stories is the person's inner determination to view their condition differently, as an experience that has occurred and from which they learned meaningful values. Inner determination surfaces and creates positive learning from the experience. It is the energy of the positive and affirming thoughts and actions that assist the healing process.

There have been other instances when people have verbally expressed determination to overcome a medically defined terminal condition. The individual may have sought practically every possible means of healing to assist in this process. Underneath it all, though, fears still linger and rise to the surface unbidden. It is these deep fearful thoughts that will invariably undo all the benefits gained. Understanding and overcoming fear is another critical step in the process to achieving lasting health and well-being.

Reducing Scarcity

Sometimes word usage has unintended consequences. This is due to the fact that the true meaning has been lost or the word has gained acceptance in another context. One example is the word "want," which actually indicates a lack of something. Webster's Dictionary defines "want" as meaning: (1) deficiency, lack, grave and extreme poverty that deprives one of the necessities of life, (2) something wanted, and (3) personal defect. How often do you hear people say, "I want this," or "I've always wanted that"? Regardless of all their seeking and striving, it is highly unlikely they will ever succeed while using that language because by using the word "want," they are actually asking for its scarcity. So when using that particular word, the individual unintentionally creates the very scarcity he or she is trying to avoid.

What words would be more appropriate to use instead? The word "want" is commonly used and accepted to mean a desire for something. If you feel you have scarcity in your life, change your language and use words like "ask for," "request," "intend" and actually imagine it happening. Even better, create the reality you intend living. Act as if you already have it. Act as if the goals are achievable. Affirm that the abundance is already within your grasp. Instead of saying and thinking that it will happen, state it as a reality. Scarcity is a state of mind. When the mind is filled with abundance, there is a resultant correlation of abundance in life.

Below is an example of how to change perceptions around scarcity. A common concern within many households relates to the lack of financial security and having sufficient funds to provide for the competing demands of daily life. My spiritual guidance suggests that you:

- give thanks for whatever finances are available;
- be grateful there is sufficient money to pay for specific financial obligations;
- continue to give thanks that there is ample money for your needs;
- focus on all the positive aspects of that money and its ability to provide staple goods; and
- affirm that there will be ongoing abundance for all needs.

When you continue affirming the positive value of money and its abundance in your life, you permeate your energy field with that intention, which eventually results in its manifestation.

By the way, there is a vast difference between desire and need. It is easy to lose sight of this difference and to categorize desires as needs when this is actually not the case. Omit the word "want" from your vocabulary and omit scarcity from your thoughts and emotions. Believe in your ability to manifest abundance for all your needs, and over time you will find that things change. You will come to see that you have more than you thought possible, and scarcity will become a thing of the past.

Often money will come from unexpected sources when you learn to trust that there is ready abundance available. A client shared a delightful story recently. She had received a parking ticket and was liable for a $50 fine. As a single mother going through a divorce settlement, the $50 fine was a substantial amount out of her weekly budget. Several days later, upon opening a Christmas card from her landlord, she found he had enclosed $50, his way of thanking her for being a model tenant. In sharing this particular story, my client also confirmed that she had the happy knack of knowing and manifesting the needed abundance in her life.

Being Consistent

There is a natural tendency in daily interactions to speak without thinking. Words often spill out automatically. It is rare to question the origin of beliefs and thoughts, let alone the real meanings of the words used regularly in conversation. People are conditioned to offer platitudes or to use expressions that are socially acceptable. Do you ever question whether what you say actually reflects your true beliefs? Do you really mean what you say? Or do your words contradict your thoughts? When there is confusion and contradiction in emotions, thoughts, words, and actions, that is what is created in your life —further confusion and contradiction. You then wonder how it is possible to change things around for the better without realizing you have actually created what you are experiencing.

This point is highly relevant to creating positive health and well-being. Being mindful of thoughts is critical to achieving real and lasting healing. Without having an awareness of the power of thought and implementing it positively on all levels, then, irrespective of whatever else you may do for self-healing, you will never fully realize your true state of wellness. Some time ago a dear friend shared her deep desires about the future of her career. A gifted body worker and healer, she had aspirations for expanding her business to include travel and teaching. As well, she spoke of her passion for making a meaningful contribution to people's lives. In the midst of this conversation, she sighed deeply and indicated that she was tired of the struggle and that a six-month break would be highly desirable. The contradiction in her thoughts, emotions, and words was apparent. She still had not achieved her goals despite her ongoing efforts. However, her words about wanting a break were actually creating what she was experiencing. All too often it is easy to say one thing, think another, and then emote and act in an entirely different manner.

Emotions originate from thoughts. Social politeness and expectations often determine what you say and do, and may not necessarily be in alignment with your real emotions and thoughts. How often do you say one thing because it is socially appropriate or it is what another person expects to hear? Do you ever give a compliment that is not genuine? It is often expedient to assert that your beliefs or thoughts are aligned with group opinion, when the opposite is actually the truth. As a social being, you are aware of what is socially correct and desirable and consequently have been taught how to behave. This means you may be placed in situations where you suppress what is actually occurring within your consciousness.

Real and lasting self-healing occurs when your thoughts, emotions, words, and actions are in alignment, work as a cohesive unit, and are positively directed—when what you say and do reflects what you actually feel and think. By doing this, you are harnessing energy into a powerful form. You combine the energies of thought, emotion, word, and action, each of them equally potent, but when aligned, they have a far greater synergistic effect. You will reap benefits at the emotional, mental, spiritual, and physical levels in unprecedented ways.

In the next chapter I will share significant strategies for manifestation I have "discovered," often through a trial-and-error process, and also via the guidance of my friends from other dimensions. However, there is nothing new in what is shared. Much of this information is ageless. It is ancient wisdom, practiced by our forebearers in their particular way. As a society, our penchant for external trappings, instant-fix solutions, and anything new and different means that it has become easy to disregard the inherent value of traditional teachings and ways.

Suggested Strategies:

Being mindful of your thoughts is critical to implementing positive change. There are several ways of achieving this:

1. Always think about what you intend to say before you express yourself.

2. Match your words and actions with your emotions and thoughts.

3. Think and speak positively at all times.

4. When a negative thought intrudes, reframe it into a positive statement.

5. Attend to often-used phrases. Eliminate them from your vocabulary.

6. Become a witness to your language. Observe the results of your thoughts and words. Then change the patterns you have created that are detrimental to your well-being.

7. Enlist the support of someone you trust to assist you in achieving consistency in language usage.

Emotional Expansion

In a previous exercise you identified the beliefs that were no longer relevant in your life. Having worked through that process, you are now ready to visualize and feel the impact of positive thoughts and emotions on your energy field.

- *Find a comfortable space. Relax your body; focus on breathing slowly and deeply. Feel the energizing breath circulate throughout your body.*

- *Hold the conscious intent that you are now going to bring universal energy into your energy field. Visualize this as a white light and feel it coming through your crown chakra, or the top of your head. This energy will fill you completely. You may experience tingling in different parts of your body.*

- *Continue breathing slowly and deeply while settling into a deeper relaxed state and feeling the energy flowing throughout.*

- *Now consciously visualize different positive thoughts and emotions on your energy field. Think of peace. What happens in your energy field? Think love, then compassion, then happiness.*

- *Allow time to feel each response within your energy field. Experiment with different positive emotions and thoughts to see whether there is a difference in your response. Do not visualize negative thoughts and emotions. The aim of this exercise is to enhance your energy field, not deplete it.*

- *Feel what is happening within your energy field. You may even see energy moving. However, you will most likely feel your heart center open and an expanded sense of love and peacefulness.*

- *Hold that feeling within and gradually return to the room you are physically in.*

When you return to full consciousness, you should be feeling very relaxed and filled with a warm, energizing feeling. This is a clear demonstration of the benefits of having only positive thoughts and emotions. These recharge your energy field and allow you to experience a stronger and calmer state of mind.

CHAPTER SIXTEEN
Manifestation Abilities

*"It is never too late to be
what you might have been."*
—George Eliot—

M anifestation is the result of intention. Whatever you experience in life is the result of your intentions. Surely it is preferable to have conscious awareness of what is happening rather than trusting to luck that everything will eventually work in your favor. When you have awareness of how reality is created, you have the power to ensure that it is one of your choosing. If, for some reason, you are dissatisfied with your reality or know that some improvement is needed, begin to implement some of the suggested strategies and exercises in this book. The strategies and exercises will not work if you only apply them for a short period. As soon as you stop and revert to former ways of thinking and feeling, you will revert to what you experienced previously. Manifestation is an ongoing process; the results you achieve are a reflection of your endeavors and intentions.

In the previous chapter an exercise demonstrated that positive thoughts and emotions create a revitalized energy field. Can you imagine what would happen to your energy field if you were to continually focus on negative thoughts? Anything that is negative will deplete and weaken your energy field. It is destructive to the energy grid.

An energy grid that is balanced consists of countless fine thread-like lines that are interconnected and parallel in several directions. What actually energizes and ensures the sensitive working of the grid are the fine golden balls that move about rapidly in all directions. Whenever a negative thought, emotion, or word is expressed, the fine thread weakens, which also impairs the natural movement of the golden balls. The process of impairment is extremely subtle and gradual. The continued expression of negativity wears down the energy grid structure so that the threads disconnect, adhere to one another, or fragment. This results in what is commonly referred to as "blocked energy" in many traditional healing modalities. When the energy is blocked, it cannot move as it is designed to. Stagnation of energy occurs, inevitably resulting in some degree of discomfort, disorder, illness, or disease.

Manifestation occurs continuously and offers you an opportunity for learning and growth. Through a process of trial and error, I have learned that:

- you create your reality;
- if you don't like your reality, you have the power to change things for the better;
- language is an extremely powerful tool for implementing meaningful change;
- manifesting involves letting go of limiting beliefs;
- manifesting is a process;
- change comes gradually;
- perseverance and belief in your ability to manifest positive change are essential to success.

It is common to think of manifestation as relating mainly to the acquisition of material goods and possessions. When you commence the process of manifesting consciously, you will find that other changes also occur. These changes relate to the inner essence that gradually modifies your self-perception and the reality you create. It is impossible to change the outer reality without significant inner changes taking place.

The reason for this is that the energy field, and its structural grid, is impacted by intentions. The positive energy created through intention has a reenergizing effect upon the energy system. Regular and persistent doses of positive thoughts and emotions create a positive surge in energies. The grid-like structure is strengthened when it receives an abundance of goodwill. There is greater strengthening of the grid structure, thereby facilitating the harmonious flow of the microscopic golden energy balls. The end result is a balanced and unified energy system. This produces uplifted emotions, enhanced mental outlook, spiritual strength, and physical wellness.

In one of his recent books Wayne Dyer explores the concept of using intention to manifest positively.[24] He offers many examples and strategies that can be successfully applied by the reader. However, the information on manifestation presented by other writers and myself is not

---

24.   Wayne Dyer. *The Power of Intention*, Hay House Inc., 2004.

new, as mentioned in the last chapter. It is merely being presented in a form that is easily understood and can be applied successfully by anyone.

As discussed in section 1, healing occurs from the outside and progresses inwardly so that tangible improvements and changes are often the last to become obvious. As you commence the process of conscious manifestation, it is likely that you will find yourself feeling less tense and have more optimism in a relatively short period of time. Personal change is a process of metamorphosis and evolves continuously. There are a number of steps that can be taken to augment the process.

1. State your intention or goal clearly from the beginning. Write it down.

2. Express your goal positively without using "want." For example, "I now have only harmonious relationships in my life."

3. Write it as if it is on its way to you or as if it is already occurring.

4. Give thanks to God, Creator, Source, or higher power of your choice for the manifestation of your intention. State your thanks as though it is already happening.

5. In some instances, it may be helpful to keep a journal to record and assess ongoing progress. If you do this, always focus on the positive and affirming. Note any learning that is occurring. Do not make judgments.

6. Have no expectations or attachment to the manner of manifestation.

7. Trust that you will learn and will be guided through the process.

8. As the manifestation unfolds or occurs, give thanks again and again.

Should you decide to manifest inner changes, the same principles apply. For example, you may choose to release self-hatred in order to come to a state of self-love. Manifestation outcomes may not necessarily be as obvious as if you were intending to find another job or car. During the process of inner change, especially, the path is bound to be uncertain, confusing, and may even seem directionless at times. This is all the more reason to have clear intent at the very outset of undertaking the process. The intention becomes the point of reference and focus when there are moments of indecision and hesitancy during the journey.

Being mindful of the language used during such a process and endeavoring to achieve consistency in this regard is an advantage. It is crucial to be determined and disciplined when undertaking a process of inner change. If you are committed to making an improvement in health and well-being, changes made in thinking around reality and your self-perception are essential. By having clear and concise intentions, you are able to systematically create the conditions for generating improvements in the desired areas.

Avoid negativity and self-doubt from percolating into thought patterns as they will undo all the hard endeavors. If there is self-doubt or negativity, it is essential to deal with this immediately. Any unconscious beliefs, patterns, and habits you hold will happily undermine your intentions and efforts. Ironically, it is usually the individual most in need of making significant changes to improve their quality of life that is the most resistant. The resistance comes from deep within and is due to long-term unconscious conditioning and deeply held fears.

Power of Positive Thought

Some straightforward ways of creating positive changes in personal reality are listed below. Over time, the cumulative effect of these changes will become evident in all areas of daily living. You will find your manifestation abilities increase when you support your intentions with positive actions. These suggestions can help create what you aspire to and offer the opportunity to enjoy what you've created.

- Begin by questioning everything. Explore avenues for learning that you previously would not contemplate. Do not judge anything, merely observe and endeavor to understand.

- Accept that there are many perspectives and beliefs. It is your responsibility to release those you hold that are limiting your growth and awareness. Accept that other people have a right to whatever beliefs they choose to hold.

- Focus attention on your thoughts. Stop negative thoughts as they come to you. You may choose to say, "Cancel that thought" and then immediately replace it with a positive thought.

- Be constantly aware of your thoughts as they surface. Then ask, "Where does this come from?" "Do I really believe, know, or feel this?" This will assist in gaining insight as to whether your thoughts are merely reflexive conditioning or are your inner truth. Remember—just because something has always been a certain way does not mean it always has to remain that way.

- Think before you speak. This slows down dialogue and creates awareness of word usage and intention. It allows you to eliminate negative thoughts and enables you to learn the art of positive expression.

- Affirm the goal to express thought in only a positive manner. Allocate a certain time for this. Begin with an hour daily and then extend it to longer periods until you are ready to embrace this way of thinking on a full-time basis.

- Make a conscious decision to speak only in a positive manner to anyone you interact with.

- Determine that whatever is spoken positively is also matched equally in thoughts and emotions. In other words, be genuine. Never make a positive statement to anyone when your feelings are the exact opposite. Doing that will ring false to the person hearing you and will not help create the desired changes.

- Be kind to yourself in all thoughts. Changing negative self-talk can be a challenge, as self-criticism is an ingrained habit for a large part of the population. Remind yourself that you are special and that others love you.

- Write lists of your attributes. You have special qualities. Focus your thoughts on what you do well and on your success stories. Remind yourself of your special talents and gifts at every opportunity.

- Positive affirmations are helpful in changing self-perception. It is vitally critical to continually monitor thoughts, beliefs, and perceptions around the self. Whenever a negative thought of self-criticism, judgment, or belittling arises, immediately dismiss it as being erroneous and then replace it with a loving and positive thought.

- If your perception of the world is pessimistic, and you always see the potential difficulties and strife in everything, it may be worthwhile enlisting the help of a trusted friend or family member. Share your desire to make specific changes and ask them to quietly monitor and support your intention. Their objectivity and sensitivity will go a long way toward assisting you through the transition process.

You choose your thoughts. Once you grasp this concept, life becomes much easier as you learn to become more selective in your thoughts and word usage. When using only positive and affirming language, you create that very same energy in life.

Learn to be Happy

This is not as impossible as it may seem. There are many magical moments in each day. Become aware and appreciative of them. There is beauty in the natural environment—in a stunning sunset, in the quietness of a forest, in the breathtaking vista seen from a mountaintop. There is joy in holding a baby, spending quality time with friends, and attending a musical performance. The list is endless.

- Begin by feeling the emotions in numerous situations and then allow the happiness to surface. If you have difficulty identifying your feelings, ask, "How do I feel?" If you are used to thinking rather than feeling, it may take some time to familiarize yourself with your true feelings. Persevere, though, as the rewards will become evident.

- Be aware of thoughts and feelings. Are they appreciative or do you continually find something to criticize? By taking inventory of the way you generally feel, you can quickly learn to stop negative reactions in midstream and from there to reframe your emotion into positive energy.

- Focus your energies on happy emotions; look for the things that create pleasure and give that "glad to be alive" feeling. Do this several times a day. Make the commitment to be happy about something or someone a minimum number of times per day. Set an initial target of twice a day and as soon as possible increase it to five; from there, consciously choose to find moments of happiness at every opportunity.

The more you focus on being happy, the more it will happen naturally. It will become an almost instinctual and normal state of emotion. There will be less negativity, criticism, and self-doubt when the energy field is filled with happy energy.

Give Gratitude

In our culture, the emphasis is on amassing material possessions and financial security. Consumerism is viewed as the means of enriching and imbuing life with meaning. Societal conditioning is such that there never seems to be enough. This is because of the general perception that external factors provide life with meaning and satisfaction.

There is more abundance in your life than you probably realize. It is easy to overlook all you have and to focus on what is lacking. Instead, give thanks for the many little and significant things that add meaning to daily life. The practice of giving gratitude adds energy to the manifestation process. Giving gratitude enhances and magnifies your intention. There are several steps involved.

- Give gratitude for what you have.
- Do this daily. Even better, do it often during the day.
- Say a quiet "thank you" prayer, listing all the things you have. Include such things as food, shelter, clothing, family, friends, health, vitality, prosperity, and so on.

- Give thanks for the nonphysical things, such as happiness, inner peace, love, creativity, and so on, as they are equally important. Remember to give thanks for the wonderful gifts and talents you possess.

- The list can be endless, but keep giving gratitude. Don't stop or miss a day. Get into the habit of being thankful for everything.

- Give thanks for the things you do not yet have but intend manifesting. Express this gratitude as though the intention is already present.

- When giving gratitude, include the words "for my highest good." There is always a higher good working for you. When you align your intentions with this divine purpose, you are able to create a truly magical reality where whatever you need is provided.

In giving gratitude, the energy of abundance is being created. An added bonus is the surprising calm and inner peace that will develop. Your world becomes filled with abundance and positive experiences. This is because you are nourishing your energy field positively. The energy grids strengthen and expand as energy is continually boosted due to the additional nourishment provided.

Ultimately, making long-lasting change for the better requires discipline, commitment, and a belief that it is possible. For a thought to become real, it must be clear, concise, and sustained over time in order for it to manifest. In reality, what you believe about the world is what you truly get!

Marvelous Manifestation

This visualization exercise will assist you to manifest your intentions. It is brief and can be used for all manifestation situations.

1. *Look at the written list or goal of your desired manifestation. Be clear in your mind about your intention.*

2. *Relax your body completely. Focus on your breath. Let go of all thoughts.*

3. When you are in a truly relaxed state, bring your consciousness to the object or outcome you intend to manifest.

4. Visualize this firmly in front of you. View it clearly as having been accomplished.

5. Now visualize the steps you have taken to achieve its manifestation. See yourself doing them effortlessly and easily.

6. Give gratitude for the manifestation of your intention. This can be in the form of a simple sentence, "Thank you, God, for bringing _____ to me."

7. Let go of the intention and visualization. Release it to a higher source. It will manifest in divine time and manner.

8. When it arrives, again give gratitude. Celebrate its arrival. This imbues positive energy to the manifestation, which carries forward to other manifestations.

CHAPTER SEVENTEEN
Energy
Flows

"Energy flows where attention goes."
—Shaman saying—

Energy of Abundance

Energy is all pervasive and ever present. Energy cannot be destroyed, though its form can be changed. As described in the previous chapter, the application of some straightforward principles of energy use has the potential to manifest a life of abundance. It is important to stress here that abundance does not necessarily pertain exclusively to gaining great wealth. Abundance in universal terms relates to ample sufficiency of all things that are for the highest good of the individual. This includes such things as abundance of sound health and vitality, joy, laughter, compassion, friendships, creativity, meaningful relationships, work, finances, peace of mind, and so on.

Your conscious mind usually has fairly fixed opinions on what constitutes abundance. This perception will always focus on what has been previously experienced and observed. Such a perception is limiting. Your inner essence, or soul, actually has a much broader perspective and understanding of abundance, of how energy works, and what is most beneficial for your spiritual growth. Learning to listen to the inner voice, or intuition, and also heeding its messages is always the first step to accessing that limitless abundance. To achieve real, meaningful, and lasting abundance, it is necessary to have the energies of word, thought, emotion, and action working together cohesively. Consistency and harmony of these is a vital component to ensuring a continual flow of abundance in your life, as was highlighted in previous chapters.

It should already be obvious that there is ample abundance available, and no one in our society need be exempt from its flow. Abundance is not just for a select few; it is meant for everyone. Everyone has the ability to access this stream. It is merely a matter of understanding how abundance manifests and then working conscientiously with that intent.

Determination Drives Intent

Have you ever had a deep desire to accomplish something special? Has that desire been so strong that it has been almost overpowering? Consequently, have you found yourself possessing determination, drive, and passion in order to achieve this particular accomplishment? This desire may have been the strivings as a youngster to gain a place in the state baseball team or it may have been the yearning to play the cello with a high degree of proficiency. No matter what the desired goal, the yearning and striving are the important factors in goal achievement.

The desire is actually the energy of intent. The determination to achieve a set goal is what drives the energy. When someone is in this state, their focus of thought, language, and emotion are directed toward a particular outcome or goal. All energies are in alignment and are focused in a positive manner. When this is the case, there is a greater likelihood of achieving the desired aim because the intensity of the combined energies is directed toward a specific outcome.

The energies become intensely focused. Even when there are moments of uncertainty or challenge, the underlying intention is not displaced in any way. If anything, the energies increase as the emphasis is on solving any problems that may interfere with the intended goal. This is because the intention is strongly chosen; there is intention that seeks fulfillment.

The energy of thought and visualization when combined produce a potent fusion of energies. When there is the added contribution of effort to thought and visualization, the resultant energy generated is even more powerful. It is important to realize that the universe does not automatically grant your wishes. You have to work for them and demonstrate your intent through practical application and dedication.

A friend would often say, "God helps those who help themselves" as he busily scurried about looking for opportunities to create an abundant life. He did more than think and visualize; he actually took every possible initiative and opportunity to expand his manifestation abilities. Unconsciously, universal energies are being harnessed to work for you whenever specific goals are stated. By directing your energies fully on your aspirations, they will manifest in a timely manner. When all your attention is given to a specific task, situation, or issue, energy will flow in that direction.

Experience is a great teacher. Most people know from experience that they are able to attain whatever is desired by hard work and determination. A general explanation for this phenomenon is that determination and hard work produces results. Intuitively, most people understand the process of harnessing and working with universal energies but may not consciously understand exactly how or why this process works so well.

Unintended Outcomes

The importance of having clarity around dreams and aspirations cannot be overstressed. How often do you hear people say, "Be careful what you ask for. You might get it"? This statement is apt. It is the language used that determines what occurs. It is easy to put the energy of abundance to work for you. However, when you desire certain material possessions or specific outcomes and put your intention into achieving those, there may be times when you are not successful despite your endeavors.

This happens for a reason. First, what is focused on may not necessarily be for your highest good and so it becomes a struggle to achieve the consciously desired intention. Second, something else oftens manifests instead. When this happens it is usually because what is manifested is what is really needed and is more appropriate than what you initially focused your intention on. The universe works in magical ways. As much as you may understand how to work with its energies, there are times when you will be reminded that you do not always consciously know what is in your best interests.

Timing

Another factor to be aware of when working to create abundance is timing. Often when working on manifesting specific outcomes, it is easy to decide on a certain time frame for manifestation to occur. Most people have the uncanny knack of seeking to control the flow of events in their life. So it is almost second nature to specify when and how the abundance is to manifest. In reality, universal consciousness does not necessarily recognize human linear time functioning. Universal time is multidimensional. Henceforth, manifestation always occurs at a time when it is most appropriate to your aspirations, needs, and spiritual growth—not necessarily when you determine is the relevant time!

Having stressed the importance of timing, there is an added bonus to manifesting through continually focusing energy positively. The more energy is focused positively for your higher good and for the higher aspirations of humanity, the more rapidly your intentions will manifest. Momentum builds up and one intention after the other is realized. Again, this is because a process of fine-tuning intentions occurs as learning takes place. A higher degree of skill evolves as you come to know and understand the manifestation process. With continuing practice, the intentions will become clear, concise, precise, and altruistic.

With altruism, the energy again expands into another form thereby accelerating the process even further. You are not experiencing life on earth for purely the attainment of selfish and self-focused interests. You have incarnated to learn and grow spiritually, and a time-honored way of doing this is to give generously to others. This is the gift of selflessness, of ensuring that all people are equally honored and respected, of knowing that your thoughts and emotions toward others are always positive, energizing, and supportive.

So far the focus of this chapter has been on the creation and manifestation of abundance and demonstrating that energy will always flow where attention is directed. The explanations indicate possibilities that exist for the creation of a harmonious environment, one in which everyone is able to access the flow of universal abundance. It would be a veritable paradise if all people and communities were able to focus energy toward the creation of a congruent and supportive way of living. Unfortunately, while there still exists a degree of unawareness of how energy works within the larger community, such aspirations will continue to be a mere ideal.

Money is Energy

In most situations it is commonplace to focus energy on the problems and struggles of daily life. Financial lack appears to be a major issue confronting a large proportion of the average population. When there is perceived lack or worry, that is exactly what occurs. The more that worry and concern impinge on the consciousness, the more obvious the signs of scarcity. The inner belief or thought reinforces and creates the actual reality.

It has been my experience and observation that when there seems to be financial scarcity the natural impulse is to try and hold on to whatever money is available. When attempting to do this, it is surprising how many unexpected demands for money suddenly crop up. Holding on to money becomes more and more difficult, especially when resistance to letting go is exerted. In this country there are many homeless people who look to the general population for some sort of aid. By giving when you think you can least afford it, you are actually creating the energy of abundance. When there is a financial contribution without expectation of receiving anything in return, that amount and often more comes back in unexpected ways. The practice of tithing works on this principle.

When money is viewed as being another form of energy, it becomes easier to understand and manage. Money arrives and is then used as needed. It has a pattern of flow. Money comes and money goes. I have learned that instead of attempting to hold on to money, it is better to bless it as it comes in and then to give another blessing as it leaves my hands. In letting go, there is a continuation of the abundance flow. While doing this I also give thanks for the ongoing abundance of money in my life.

Blocking Abundance

A common blockage to receiving the flow of abundance is being unable or unwilling to accept. If you have difficulty in accepting compliments or the generosity of others, your lack of receptivity blocks whatever is waiting to flow to you. Graciously accept compliments without any negative thoughts intruding. Learn to accept kind offers of assistance and support, even when they are not really needed, as they further accelerate the flow of abundance. People love to share their skills, time, and abundance. Ultimately, you have to be open and receptive in order to receive. It's as simple as that!

In many instances when there is scarcity in your life, there may be an inherent and subconscious belief of unworthiness. This belief says, "I don't deserve any better." This belief may relate to financial status, relationships, and employment opportunities, for example. Again, such beliefs need to be seriously examined, understood, and then gradually turned around into supportive and affirming beliefs.

When an individual focuses on the lack of a significant relationship in his or her life, that is what actually happens. When a parent criticizes a child regarding perceived imperfections and misdemeanors, that child will then respond accordingly. When a medical condition causes concern, that medical condition will predominate in a person's planning and living arrangements. There will be a focus on the symptoms, and eventually those symptoms will be present constantly and in time will worsen. Whatever you perceive and focus your time and energy on is what ultimately happens. This is because energy flows where attention goes!

A client, a mother of two young children, shared her story about healing a debilitating back condition. She found her back was weakening. Doctors prescribed pain relief medication and physiotherapy exercises. Surprisingly, instead of getting better, she found that the more she complied with the specialists' directives, the weaker she became. Even carrying the shopping bags from the car to the house became a nightmarish effort. One day she decided that enough was enough—being infirm was not suiting her needs and certainly did not fit in with her long-term plans. That decision was the turning point. She decided that she was no longer in pain, and with that decision, her back slowly and steadily regained its strength and former flexibility. When I met her, she exhibited no sign of back discomfort or disability.

Globally we live in a time of uncertainty and change. World events impinge upon your consciousness and impact whatever happens daily. Incidents occurring elsewhere affect you. Conversely, whatever happens on an individual level also affects what happens within the wider community and globally. If you truly desire to create improvement and change, then with conscious intent you can begin to implement positive outcomes. The more this happens, the more your energy field expands. You have the power to create a world that is safe. You have the ability to manifest harmony and peace. Whatever your specific intention in this regard, it is important to always focus on creating the changes within yourself initially. Focus the intent (energy) on manifesting inner peace and awareness. Focus the energies to create the reality that is for your highest good, and in time the benefits will flow outwardly to other people. The more you consciously do this, the greater the returns. By focusing your energies positively and creatively, you will, like an investment banker, continue to build up the value of your stocks, all of which will enhance your quality of life.

Suggested Strategies

In implementing the following suggestions, you will have a clearer indication of exactly how you are creating whatever happens in your life. Once you begin to understand your role in creating events, you are able to mindfully create enhanced outcomes in every way.

- Listen to what you say. Is your disposition usually positive? Or are you mostly negative in thoughts and language?

- Look for patterns in negative thinking and expression. Do you hold certain beliefs about yourself or about life? If so, follow the exercises outlined in chapter 14.

- Write down the significant things that happen to you over a two- to four-week period. Reflect on thoughts and language used prior to incidents or issues. Is there a connection?

- Assess your family's attitudes toward health, wealth, and life in general. How many of these have you unconsciously absorbed into your reality? Are you willing to change any that are not serving you positively?

- Write a list of your beliefs and feelings around money. This will reveal clearly whatever you are manifesting in terms of financial abundance or scarcity.

CHAPTER EIGHTEEN
Understanding and Overcoming Fear

"If you feel safe within yourself,
there is no fear of the world around you."
—Unknown Source—

It has been said that there are only two emotions, love and fear. It is also claimed that the emotion of love in its true sense involves the absence of fear. Fear is nebulous. Some fears are understood, acknowledged, and lived with. Other fears are subconscious; they are not usually acknowledged, but continue to impact insidiously upon decisions and actions taken throughout your life journey. Fear is inculcated into beliefs and perceptions from very early in life. It is reinforced in countless daily interactions and is widespread globally through shared perceptions of other cultures and world events. Fear has become a constant companion in practically all cultures.

Fear is energy. It is palpable and emanates outward from its source. This is most evident when you are in the presence of someone who is experiencing extreme fear. It is very easy for that person's fear to permeate the energy fields of people he or she interacts with. In a relatively short space of time the fear spreads—maybe not initially or as intensely—but it nevertheless becomes a shared reality. It is spread in much the same way as a contagious disease or virus is—from one person to the next. The only difference is that fear is a deep-seated mental and emotional response and is usually based on irrational beliefs.

Fear exists on the mental, emotional, and spiritual levels and is usually expressed at the physical level in terms of responses to situations. Fear, like other forms of negativity, has a damaging effect on the energy grid. It too distorts, fractures, and weakens the grid structure. It can be likened to a heavy mass that rests within a space of lightness. The contrast is extreme. The heavy (and dark) mass is energy and has weight. This weight suffocates the light and clear energy that is contained within the energy field, resulting in some degree of energy imbalance.

In most instances people become accepting of the fears they hold, believing it is normal to have such fears. This is because conditioning has taught us that the world is not a safe place to live. In theory, infants should be protected from the possible evils of the world by those responsible for their upbringing. However, it must be acknowledged that adults too are a product of their upbringing and therefore perpetuate their beliefs and perspectives on their progeny. Through this process you come to have awareness that the world is not safe and that you need to be careful when venturing away from your point of safety. Some common fears are:

- it is not safe to walk alone in the dark,
- it is not safe to leave the doors and windows in your home unlocked,
- travel to overseas countries is risky, and
- other people cannot be trusted.

A paradigm is created, one in which it is believed that you can survive only by viewing unknown and unfamiliar people, issues, and situations with suspicion. It is all too easy to view the world through fear-colored glasses.

A couple of years ago, I encountered a delightful elderly woman at a photo specialty shop. We engaged in pleasantries while waiting to be served, and during the conversation she commented that the world was no longer a safe place. My response was to ask what she meant by her statement. In reply she asserted that her home was likely to be burglarized, and because of this she no longer felt safe living there. Her belief around this was most likely contributed to by the numerous media reports on home invasions occurring in the city where we lived. Or it may have been created by the fact that she was no longer young and so felt vulnerable. When questioned further she admitted that she had never been the victim of a burglary. My response was that we attract into our lives whatever we fear. What I shared was a reminder that she really had nothing to fear and that she was being fooled into believing something that was not necessarily real for her.

The energy of fear will always fester and proliferate while attention is focused on it. Remember, energy flows where attention goes! Media reporting mainly focuses on disasters, misfortunes, and mishaps. Good news stories only make up a very small percentage of what is reported daily. As a society, we have become conditioned and expect to hear only bad news.

There is a saying in metaphysical circles that what you fear is what you attract into your life. The form it takes may not necessarily be as anticipated, but it will come in some related manner so you can learn from the experiences and ultimately learn to overcome those fears. The person who fears for their safety when traveling will most likely have challenging travel experiences. These fears will only be overcome when the individual chooses to confront the fears and deal with them in an appropriate manner. A person who fears the loss of a relationship will subconsciously, and sometimes consciously, be looking for signs that the relationship is not working. That creates an energy of mistrust and uncertainty. Their partner will feel that lack of trust, become weary of dealing with emotional responses, and is then more likely to react accordingly. This is somewhat like the self-fulfilling prophecy where a person believes something and what is believed (or feared) ends up occurring.

Fear limits your ability to truly enjoy the beautiful life you are meant to live. It is easy to become accepting of the fears you hold and to allow them to restrict life adventures. This means you eventually accept the limitations that certain fears impose upon your choices. In many instances, fears are so deeply embedded that there is no consciousness around them. These too restrict and impinge deeply upon your opportunities to truly grow as a unique being.

Becoming aware of your fears, both conscious and subconscious, is necessary to understanding and releasing them. Many skilled and knowledgeable people who have studied phobias and fears extensively have already written a great deal about this subject. Through personal experiences and in working with clients I have observed:

1. There is great value in systematically addressing fears, in recognizing them through cognitive processing and then analyzing them. Such an approach involves thinking and rationalizing, which assists greatly in reaching understanding. However, having understanding is only the beginning of the process.

2. It is necessary to engage fully in the emotional aspect as well as having cognitive understanding in order for meaningful healing to occur.

3. Fear has an emotional component, and for fear to be healed, it must involve the release of emotional reactions and beliefs.

There are countless strategies that can be used to overcome fears. In most instances each will require patience, courage, and belief in your ability to create change. Once you embark on a journey of releasing fears, they have the knack of making their presence known, one after the other. It is similar to peeling an onion. There is layer upon layer that is waiting and ready to be peeled away.

Writing as a Tool

One of my favorite strategies is to use writing as a tool in the healing process. These steps will assist you to bring to the surface conscious and some subconscious fears. Identification of fears is necessary before healing can occur.

- Write a list of fears that you hold. Initially, most of what is listed will be the obvious fears. This may include fear of heights, spiders, not being in control, walking alone after dark, sleeping in the dark, having a terminal disease or condition, and losing a loved one.

- With each fear identified ask, "Is there a deeper fear lurking beneath this?" The reason for asking this is that you are endeavoring to bring to your awareness a list of all fears you hold, not merely the obvious ones.

- Some fears may relate to others. For example, a fear of the dark could also be linked to a fear of not being able to see clearly. Identify the fears that are linked and group them together.

- Ask, "How would I feel if this fear actually happens?" of each identified fear. Jot down your immediate emotional response. This will probably be a word or phrase only.

- Describe in writing, step by step, exactly what would happen in each specific situation. In most instances, the worst-case scenario may be grim but not necessarily as disastrous as feared. You will also discover baseless fears when undertaking this exercise.

- Assess the validity of each fear you have dissected and analyzed. How real is the fear? Is it in your mind? How strong is your emotional reaction? Do you hold the fear due to conditioning or a belief? Is it likely to happen now or in the distant future? Realistically appraise each fear listed. Many, if not most, will be found lacking in substance.

- Are there any fears you can resolve by taking some positive steps? Identify those and then act on them.

It might be worth mentioning that you possess the skills to deal with whatever happens in life and the strength and ability to come to a state of acceptance around whatever challenging issues arise. Once this insight is understood, there is greater acceptance of whatever may possibly happen, and with that comes peace of mind. There is also the strong possibility that what is feared is unlikely to ever happen or in the manner anticipated. Going through a process of examination allows that recognition, and from there the fear diminishes. It loses its power to paralyze you mentally and emotionally.

Subconscious Fears

It is possible to take positive steps in overcoming subconscious fears. At different times there may be subconscious fears that percolate to the surface of your consciousness. As these arise, a similar process of analysis is necessary to achieve understanding of the inherent nature of the fear. From there it is a matter of again working through the fear so that its power fades.

An example of this is someone I know who exhibits a fear of change. This fear becomes apparent when discussion arises around holiday travel and new employment opportunities. Her response is to articulate clearly her justification for remaining in the same job, despite the fact that she is unhappy with practically every aspect of her employment. Similarly when holiday travel arrangements are discussed, she maintains the perfect holiday is staying in her hometown. This person would deny having any fear. Instead she maintains she does not like change or uncertainty in her life.

Not being a psychologist by trade, it is not for me to say specifically what is the reason for her aversion to, or fear of, change. However, knowing her reasonably well, this aversion is probably related to a period of unsettlement that she experienced as a young child. If at some stage she allows her subconscious fears around change to surface, it would provide an opportunity to explore her deeply held beliefs and perceptions around feeling safe. It would most likely result in greater emotional empowerment.

Whenever you hold a strong conviction about some aspect of your life, it is likely there is an underlying fear driving that conviction. It is easy to assert that things are the way they are and that change is impossible. Yet most people love to dream of the wonderful changes they would like to have in their lives. It is easy to dream of achieving success and of doing something remarkably worthwhile, as most people aspire to. In most instances such dreams are not realized because of an underlying fear of failure or even of achieving success. Another commonly held fear is that of being perceived as different from mainstream society. Individuals generally crave approval from family, friends, and peers. These fears limit the inner creativity and initiative that are often screaming out for release. Then, too, there is the inherent fear of not being good enough, not smart enough, not worthy enough, and so on.

Whatever fear holds you back is worthy of your time and attention. For example, if you yearn to become a graphic designer (or something else) but are convinced that you lack sufficient creative talent, then:

1. Ask yourself why you hold this belief. Where did it originate? How realistic is this perception? What occurred in your earlier years to create this belief?

2. Continue delving into your conscious and subconscious minds to find the reason for any unreasonable fears you hold as truth.

3. Examine your life for incidents and events that have helped shape your perceptions about yourself and your place in the world.

4. Assess whether they have created deep fears within you.

5. Observe how those fears have shaped your life and how they have placed limitations upon your life choices.

6. Continue asking, "Why do I believe this?" "What is the truth of this?"

7. Assess whether they have any relevance to your current situation.

Become the Witness

Become the observer, or witness, of your fear reactions and beliefs. As an observer you have no emotional attachment. You can see with greater clarity what is actually happening; you observe your thinking process and the related emotions. Observing allows you to be free of any bias. It enables you to understand with greater insight the how, when, where, and why of the fear.

1. Ask what events or people shaped this fear (how).
2. Ask at what time in your life were you first aware of this fear and in what situation does it still arise (when).
3. Ask about the situation or location and how it has impacted on you (where).
4. Ask the reason for the fear (why).

Again, it may be helpful to write down what is observed, as often the important minute details can be lost when left to memory. Having a written record of observations provides a record of progress and may be useful when other fears percolate to the surface at another time. Often one fear is linked to another, and it is only by working through them as they clamor for attention that their deeper meaning can be accessed. In many ways a process such as this reminds me of detective novels I used to read enthusiastically. Detectives follow up on whatever clues appear, however random they may seem, and through a process of trial and error, deduction, and often sheer instinct, they are able to solve the mystery.

Being an observer is one practical way of gaining deeper understanding of whatever fear is operating. Once there is understanding, in most instances there is an awareness of the irrationality of the fear. Fears tend to be irrational, though they have the power to immobilize you from living your truth. With understanding comes release. The fear loses its power and impetus, especially when this is combined with positive intent and thinking. Changing your self-talk is empowering, and, when armed with determination to affirm only positive and loving thoughts, can turn fear into courage.

Taking small positive steps to overturn the fear may also be useful once the observation phase has been implemented. One small step at a time ultimately results in many steps being taken, which will result in healing old emotions. Whatever strategy is used should be in alignment with the fear that has surfaced and should not place you at any risk. The intention is to reduce and eventually eliminate the fear, not to create further stress.

Meditation As A Tool

Meditation is a powerful tool and can be used to recognize and overcome fears. My experience has been that it is important to be familiar and comfortable with the meditation process before this tool can be utilized. There have been instances when I've had awareness of a fear but have been uncertain about its origin. In seeking to absolve the fear from my system, my spiritual guides have acceded to my requests to have it revealed. This is not a process I would ever recommend for a beginning meditator. Sometimes the information shown is very subtle. It is a matter of understanding what has been revealed and then taking action to release the fear.

One significant benefit of meditation, however, is that it calms the mind and emotions. Whatever fears you carry seem less momentous when meditation is undertaken regularly. Worry and stress fade away when you allow yourself to relax totally. When the meditation is finished, the feeling of relaxation carries through into the day's activities.

My spiritual guides have always insisted on the importance of undertaking daily reflection practice or meditation. Even for people who insist that meditation is too difficult, there are other worthwhile activities and strategies that can be utilized to relax the mind, such as listening to gentle music, jogging, painting, and so on. The important thing is to take time to relax, to give time to being in the moment, and letting go of worry. Schedule time on a daily basis for this. It may mean having to forego watching the news or some other favorite television show or possibly even getting up fifteen minutes earlier each morning. Making the effort to incorporate time for yourself every day, in which you are able to quietly reflect and just be, will prove worthwhile within a few months of starting such a regime. Having a daily routine for reflection practice or meditation assists in minimizing and releasing worries and fears.

Spiritual Principles

There are several spiritual principles involved around the issue of fear conditioning that are worth keeping in mind.

1. What you fear is what you attract into your life. This is a universal law and is designed to help you overcome whatever is feared. If you fear speaking in public, situations will arise that necessitate speaking to others, whether it be to groups, family, or people in authority. Once that fear has been overcome, there will be fewer similar challenges occurring in that particular regard.

2. Fear is an emotion and, as such, has energy. This energy is emitted through your energy field and attracts other people who hold similar energy, resulting in a larger pool of fear. Eventually this spills outward as it increases. It then creates a reality of fear where incidents and events affirm the reason for the fear. In other words, it eventually becomes a self-fulfilling cycle.

3. What you think, you create. If you think your neighbors are untrustworthy, then regardless of whatever actions they may take, those actions will be construed as being dishonest. If you perceive the leader of a country to be bad, the evidence will unfold to support that perception. If, through the media information you absorb, you know that the world is not a safe place, your daily experiences will reinforce that knowing.

4. Everyone is your mirror. What you see in others is what you hold within. When you see intolerance in someone, it is because you hold intolerance within and recognize that aspect of yourself in another. You might be inclined to deny this especially when you perceive a negative trait in someone that you would never believe possible in yourself. The people who come into your life do so for a reason and are your best teachers, especially those who really challenge you the most, for they mirror many behaviors and characteristics that you wish to deny or not deal with.

5. As a spirit being having a human experience, you are part of the One, as is everyone else. So when you judge another, you also

judge yourself. Taking that further, when you hurt another, you also hurt yourself, and so on. The myth of separation from the Creator has resulted in this sense of alienation and aloneness. It has become acceptable to view others as different. They are judged by their skin color, race, creed, and so on. Instead of rejoicing in the similarities, it is common to focus on the differences. Fear and negativity support the contention that we are not One in spirit. Rather, they create further alienation within the individual.

Fear is part of the human condition, and you have incarnated to learn from it. Suppressing fear does not bring about healing, nor will it disappear because it is ignored. I have focused attention on how fear perpetuates and the steps that can be taken to reduce and eventually release its power. Releasing deep-seated fears is another of life's journeys. It is an individual journey that ultimately leads to a feeling of inner peace and security. Once that is attained, nothing can take it away.

The more you practice being loving and compassionate in thoughts and gestures, the less room there is within your energy field for fear to predominate. With continual striving toward the state of compassion and love, there can be no room for fear to ferment. When this is the intent, there will come the day when there is an awareness of a feeling of inner safeness. When this happens there is an understanding that nothing in the external reality can ever hurt you.

Flying Fearlessly

This visualization is designed to assist the release of any particular fear you may hold. Also included are steps to replace the fear with love, thereby creating a feeling of inner safety. In order to maximize the benefits of this visualization, I recommend that you initially follow the strategies suggested earlier in this chapter for identifying and understanding your fears.

1. *Find a quiet, comfortable space. Sit with your feet flat on the floor and your arms resting in your lap, palms upward.*

2. *Focus on your breath. Breathe slowly and deeply.*

3. When in a relaxed state, concentrate on a fear you have identified and are ready to release.

4. Observe this fear. Where does it sit in your body? Can you feel it in your energy field? When you are in a totally relaxed state, you will have a sense of where it is sitting and the feelings you have around it.

5. Hold the mental image of where the fear is located. Visualize the mass of fear being surrounded by golden light. You may even be able to "see" the energy grid where the fear is held. If you are unable to visualize this, pretend it is happening. Now the fear is encapsulated with golden light and you are ready to move it.

6. Steadily, using the power of your mind, see the fear being released out of your body and right out of your energy field. You may even be able to see what is happening in the energy grid as the fear exits. Know that it is being released to a higher power.

7. As you do this, say a short prayer of thanks. "I release this fear of _____ with love. I release it to a higher power. I thank the fear for showing me _____."

8. As you feel the release, continue to focus on your breathing. You may feel the release as a gentle tingling in the area, or you may feel a definite pulling sensation. Both are perfectly normal. Once the release has occurred, you will most likely experience a feeling of lightness in the area where the fear was stored.

9. Now focus on the area from which the fear has been released. Visualize golden light streaming into your body to this space. Feel it filling the space previously occupied by the fear mass. See the energy grid being restored to a state of balance.

10. When you are ready, make a statement of affirmation. "I now feel love where there was fear. In this state of love, I am safe and strong. I am love." This affirmation can be used any time you experience a fear reaction.

11. Feel your inner quiet and calm. Remain there for as long as you choose. When ready, bring your awareness back to the room.

Section	**SPIRITUAL**
Three	**PRINCIPLES**

CHAPTER NINETEEN
A Spiritual Perspective

Not I, nor anyone else can travel that road for you.
You must travel it by yourself.
It is not far; it is within reach.
Perhaps you have been on it since you were born,
and did not know.
Perhaps it is everywhere—on water and land.
—Walt Whitman—

It is important to integrate some spiritual practice into daily life for real and lasting healing to occur. I am not referring to attendance at church or participation in bible-reading groups on a regular basis. Living a spiritual life permeates all aspects of life and inner being, irrespective of where you are, what you are doing, or what is occurring.

There is a quandary around defining or explaining what living a spiritual life signifies. For some people it is likely there is an instant thought that this relates to religion or religious beliefs. That is not the intention, nor the case, as all that is shared in this book comes largely from my perceptions, experiences, and learning. My seeking has largely been from within, and this is where a vast amount of my knowing originates. What is acknowledged, however, is that the majority of religions and beliefs share similar values and messages regarding how we are to live a life of seeking and striving. You will find aspects of these values and messages contained within these pages, as they are inherent to spiritual growth and awareness, regardless of doctrine or tenet.

The underlying emphasis in this book so far has been about healing the energy grid within the larger energy field. The importance of achieving balance within the energy field has been stressed. There is an additional benefit in having a balanced energy field. There are significant changes occurring as blockages are released and as intention is changed from negative to positive. The energy that created distortion and fracturing within the energy grid is released and is replaced with light energy. The more that is released, the more light fills the energy field. Spiritual teachings state that enlightenment is the ultimate goal of spiritual striving. I believe that energetically the process of enlightenment involves releasing all stored blockages, thereby enabling the body to hold more light.

Most people strive to make sense of their lives and the world in general. Usually, when faced with a trauma or crisis situation, there is no choice but to delve deeper into the meaning of life. It would be realistic to assert that, generally, at some time in everyone's life comes a point when there is questioning around the meaning and purpose of life. For some people, this seeking comes early in life; for others it does not occur until their departure is imminent.

In my line of work it is common for clients to share their experiences. Often there is great confusion, uncertainty, and pain around life issues and emotions they have encountered. At other times they seek healing for pain while stating there is something greater than them, outside their normal experiences, that guides their seeking. They acknowledge an unseen force that is always there when they need help. More and more I see people openly sharing their otherworld experiences. As a universal humanity, it seems we are becoming increasingly aware of something outside ourselves, something that drives us to look at the unseen, to examine the many layers of reality and in that process to gain real understanding of our origins and purpose.

Most people aspire to living a spiritual life though not everyone would express it in such terms. There are times when I have had the pleasure of knowing delightfully warm and generous people who would not profess to be spiritually inclined, yet when listening to their words and observing their demeanor and behaviors, it is patently obvious that their lives are based upon spiritual truths and principles. They have an inherent belief in the goodness within all beings, are positive and uplifting in personality and nature, and accept that life is what it is.

In earlier chapters the concept of energy was explored at length. Along with this, the benefits of thinking positively, using affirming language and reducing negativity in life in order to achieve healing and well-being were stressed. This section of the book, however, concentrates on the process of inner seeking in the healing process, and relating the inner journey to the manner in which life can be lived meaningfully and with clarity.

Whatever energy you create influences all aspects of your life and all levels of functioning. The spiritual cannot be separated from the physical, emotional, or mental levels at which you operate. To omit the spiritual aspect is to live as though functioning on three-quarters capacity. To my way of thinking, it is somewhat like taking a car to the mechanic and asking him for a tune-up of the engine, but requesting that he complete only three-quarters of the tune-up.

In life there is always choice (free will), and some people appear to be perfectly happy without the need to recognize and acknowledge their spiritual self. There will come a time, however, when this lack in their life results in situations and conditions for which they will not be fully prepared nor able to deal with easily. When the individual is receptive to their inner essence and works with it, there is greater opportunity for dealing with the diverse vagaries of life's journey, resulting in reduced stress. In addition, it is likely that the individual will have greater inner peace and a sense of real purpose.

It is likely that practically every reader of this book has had an unusual, unexplainable, or paranormal experience at some time in his or her life. Most often these experiences or encounters leave the individual feeling confused and uncertain. "Did I really see what I thought I saw?" "No one would ever believe me if I told them about this." "I know what I felt and saw, but how can I explain it?" These are only some of the common reactions to incidents that occur outside normal expectations and paradigms. My clients share many of their unusual experiences, often expressing concern that they're unable to be more open publicly about such things.

As a culture we have become so conditioned to believe that scientific reasoning and application are the status quo and that all phenomena and experiences must fit into and adhere to the scientific mold. When unexplainable things happen, there is an immediate endeavor to justify and analyze them so that they can be subsumed into daily existence in a rational way. Fortunately the world of spirit doesn't necessarily work according to currently held scientific dogmas and theories!

The first step toward becoming more spiritually aware is to seek. That is all. Seeking spiritual truth can be likened to holding a key in hand and advancing toward a door that is locked. It is the willingness to let go of preconceived ideas and expectations that will lead you to the door where you will, with ease, insert the key and unlock the door. Only you hold the key to unlocking the door to your inner essence or soul. It is the predisposition to do so that is the critical ingredient. The door cannot be unlocked until you are ready to venture further. You may feel that such a venture is exciting and will embrace it with fervor and enthusiasm. Or you may find yourself being led, often reluctantly, to the door, and it is with hesitation that each little step forward is taken. This hesitation is due to the conscious mind and its attitude to all things spiritual and unseen.

When there is conscious resistance to inner spiritual questing, it is often the soul that is actually urging and encouraging the undertaking of such a venture. This in turn leads to emotional and mental conflict because of conscious will and resistance. You may well see the signs that are placed in your path but are reluctant to accept and embrace a new way of seeing and living. On a conscious level, this resistance indicates the presence of fear and may relate to fear of change, fear of being viewed differently, and fear of risk taking.

Once the door is unlocked, it opens slowly, revealing its mystical energies and phenomena. What happens next is personal; the spiritual journey is your unique experience. Through this experience you will witness the world in new, different, and exciting ways. Your perceptions and experiences will not be the same as mine, your neighbor's, or that of anyone else. It will become evident along the way, however, that there are many commonly shared concepts and truths. That is inevitable.

There is a misperception held by some people within our communities that only churchgoers and those having a specific religious faith can find the way to God or to salvation. In the mid '90s, I was fortunate to attend a talk given by the Dalai Lama to a small audience of about twelve hundred people. His discourse roamed over a vast range of topics, but one analogy he shared serves as a reminder of the need for acceptance and tolerance of people holding differing perspectives and beliefs.

The Dalai Lama asked us to imagine that a new restaurant had opened in our locality. Its menu was a single offering only, a dish that was exquisite, mouth-watering, and tantalizing. This specific menu offering was available for lunch and dinner, seven days a week for months and months endlessly. Imagine being a regular diner at this restaurant. Realistically there is no guarantee that your palate will savor or enjoy the exquisite meal, as it may not even be to your taste. As it is the only option available, culinary boredom will invariably result. There would also be an accompanying lack of appreciation of its exquisiteness.

It must be remembered though that there is absolutely nothing wrong with this menu offering. Its only limitation is lack of choice, which diners are not accustomed to experiencing. It is the same with belief systems. The Dalai Lama pointed out that Islam is the faith that appeals to some people, Catholicism is a more suitable faith system for others, while Hinduism feels right for certain populations. In the Dalai Lama's particular instance, obviously Buddhism is the philosophy that resonates for him. It is his best spiritual match.

Underlying his delightful analogy, however, is the recognition and acceptance that there are many paths available, all leading to the Creator. There is no one faith, religion, or belief that is better than another. There is no right or wrong choice when you align yourself with a particular belief system. Whatever belief you choose to align with has a resonance for you, and it becomes your vehicle for seeking deeper meaning to life.

Recently I attended a palliative training workshop at which a panel of spiritual leaders shared information about their respective faiths. This panel comprised a diversity of beliefs, including Jewish, Roman Catholic, Navajo, Hopi, Anglican, Jesus Christ of Latter Day Saints, and others. It was heartening to hear their differing perspectives while observing their calm acceptance and support of the differing doctrines. While there were certainly differences, it became apparent that many similarities were shared.

Mahatma Gandhi stated it thus: "The various religions are like different roads converging on the same point. What difference does it make if we follow different routes, provided we arrive at the same destination?"

Ultimately, when seeking, the intention is to reconnect with a greater divine power. This is the common reason for all religions and faiths. Along with this, there is the implicit understanding that it is not for you to judge the respective merits of belief systems different from one that you may choose. As there is no right or wrong choice when it comes to spiritual belief systems, surely there cannot be any reason to criticize or judge another's faith. There can be no justification for exhibiting intolerance and rejection of another's devotional practices. However, in our world there is a strong history of religious intolerances, along with many wars carried out in the name of religious righteousness. The history of the last couple of thousand years is testimony to this statement. Yet, because it has been that way for so long does not mean it has to continue in the same vein.

Humanity is now at the brink of a new era in consciousness. This will be an era in which preconceptions, prejudices, and intolerances can be released and healed. This is a unique opportunity in our global history for all people to open their hearts to one another with compassion and acceptance. A true commitment to world peace and harmony can only be achieved when there is acceptance, tolerance, and support for the diversity of beliefs that exist.

In terms of spirituality, it seems that the word "spiritual" is often perceived as a negative belief or practice and is not accepted by some religious adherents, as it is not espoused within their religious tenets. To some people the word may imply paranormal experiences, such as ouija board activities, holding séances, and having visitations from ghosts and poltergeists that are often scary and extreme. That is not what spirituality in its true sense means.

According to the Dalai Lama, there is a distinction between religion and spirituality. Religion contains teachings, rituals, prayer, dogma, and so on, whereas spirituality is "concerned with those qualities of the human spirit—such as love and compassion, patience, tolerance, forgiveness, contentment, a sense of responsibility, a sense of harmony—which bring happiness to both self and others . . . . This is why I sometimes say that religion is something we can perhaps do without. What we cannot do without are these basic spiritual qualities."[25]

A person who is seeking spiritual enlightenment looks deeply within to find the meaning of life. It is not something that is external to the individual. Spiritual people find their connection with a higher divine source in a way that is uniquely meaningful to them. During this process they come to acknowledge a greatly expanded view of creation and reality that is not necessarily aligned with the beliefs of many religions. They endeavor to imbue their lives with the qualities of compassion, tolerance, acceptance, service, nonjudgment, and other positive attributes in all aspects of daily life. For most, there is an acceptance and

---

25. Dalai Lama. *Ancient Wisdom, Modern World*, Little, Brown and Company, 1999.

connection with other spirit beings, including spirit guides and angels that come to the earth plane to be of assistance.

This section of the book explores some core spiritual principles that are essential to healing. When discussing healing, it is always in relation to healing of the self. This is for a specific reason. A spiritual journey is an individual passage. It requires intense inner focus and commitment and cannot be undertaken for someone else. Healing the self on a spiritual level sets in place an opportunity for healing on every other level, including the physical body. A great deal of pain and many wounds are spiritual in origin though they may manifest as otherwise.

One of the ingredients essential for successful healing is that of living a life based on love. This does not refer to love involving emotional attachment or love that is conditional. Rather, it is universal and humanitarian love and is the most potent force in all creation. Love is the essence of who you are. Recognizing this and integrating the energy of universal love fully into your being will result in healing on all levels.

In the following chapters, the principles of love, forgiveness, nonattachment, letting go of expectations, having acceptance, and being in the moment will be fully explored. There are examples explaining how these principles can be applied meaningfully in daily activities. By implementing changes in behavior, language, and intention, it gradually becomes easier to feel connected to a higher source and to manifest a reality that is in alignment with your soul's purpose. When this happens, healing on the spiritual level occurs and a new and meaningful level of empowerment results. From this comes the opportunity to truly live the life that is waiting for you, and not necessarily the one that you have planned!

Spirit Guides

I often hear people comment that they would like to know more about their guardian angel or spirit guides. The ability to communicate with beings from another dimension is also desired. The reasons for this are many. Mostly, though, there is a yearning to know more, to seek guidance, and to gain an understanding of whatever exists beyond the known physical reality.

The ability to communicate with spirit guides is possible for everyone. I have listed a number of steps that can be applied to facilitate this process. There is a reason for referring to this as a process. Spirits communicate in countless ways, most of which are extremely subtle. It is a matter of recognizing the messages or signs that are given. With practice this becomes easier.

- State the intention that you are ready to communicate with your spirit guides.

- Ask your spirit guides to communicate with you. Ask for messages that are for your highest good and that provide assistance on your spiritual path.

- Your guides have probably been communicating with you all along, though that does not mean you have been listening. By stating your intention, you are indicating your willingness to listen and receive.

- Allow spirit the opportunity to be heard. This involves meditating regularly, as well as making other quiet times available.

- During meditation or other quiet times, you may feel a warm, tingling sensation alongside your body. Pay attention to this. It may be your guides communicating with you or demonstrating their presence.

- Spirit messages may come as an instant knowing of something. They may arrive as a strong sense of emotional awareness around some issue. Or you may even hear words clearly articulated, though softly spoken.

- Messages from spirit guides are never negative. Your spirit guides will never judge or criticize. They are supportive and encourage your spiritual growth. If you should receive a message that is negative, tell the spirit to leave you. Only accept messages that are positive and those you intuitively feel are for your highest good.

Spirit guides communicate in many different ways. Here are some commonly used means:

- Words in a book will seemingly "jump out" at you.

- You hear a song title that is pertinent to whatever is happening in your life.
- Spirit will give you a message through the words of different people.
- There will be several coincidences with the same meaning.
- In the morning as you awaken, just before regaining full consciousness, you may receive a message.
- Messages come in dreams, usually in lucid dreaming where there is clarity and cohesiveness.
- Messages are continually sent via Mother Nature. The presence of animals, birds, and insects should always be viewed as another likely communication.
- Communicate with your spirit guides as though you were conversing with a close friend. Share your concerns, desires, and so on. Ask for guidance and suggestions. They will come in subtle ways at first. With practice, you will come to recognize their valuable contribution to your life.

CHAPTER TWENTY
Trusting Self

"Nothing we ever imagined is beyond our power,
only beyond our present self-knowledge."
—Theodore Rozak—

In endeavoring to find meaning in life, it is easy to look to others to define who you are and to determine what is important. Early conditioning creates the belief that other people are able to provide the answers, regardless of whether you are seeking healing on a physical or any other level. If ever there is a time when it is possible for you to become empowered to take responsibility for your health and wellness, that time is now. You have two important resources available for this.

First, whatever information you seek is readily available. There is abundant information available on all aspects of health. It is a matter of making time to research, ask questions, and become better informed as to possible options. Second, you are able to exert free will in the treatment of your health and wellness. There are far more choices available than there were fifty years ago. Accept and acknowledge that your health and well-being are your responsibility. Maintain that perspective. Always trust your instinctual knowing around your body and its needs.

This chapter explains how you can become empowered in your quest for wellness. As mentioned earlier, looking to others to take responsibility for whatever happens in your life results in disempowerment on all levels. In addition, your energy field is also compromised. Becoming empowered involves learning to trust your instinctual or inner knowing, allowing yourself to be guided, and to always seek whatever is for your highest good. Your goal in self-healing is to create a strong and balanced energy grid. As you are already beginning to understand, this is a steady and complex process. The principles shared in this chapter are important to healing and creating wellness and will further enhance the healing already occurring within your energy field.

Nothing ever happens by chance. I have come to value the subtle ways messages are sent by spirit guides. In early 2003, a friend shared her feelings of despondency. Apparently she had read a book on the chakra system. There was information relating to each chakra center and signs indicated where dysfunction exists. She read the book with the intention of acquiring greater knowledge and spiritual insight. Instead, subjectively, she labeled her strivings as a failure due to what she read and interpreted. At that instant, it was as if a lightbulb switched on inside my head. Encapsulated within a nanosecond of time was a profound insight. It is unlikely I'll be able to do justice in explaining that insight, but I will try to give a sketchy outline.

The understanding that the search for meaning lies within, and not from an external source, became more powerful than ever. Added to this was the knowing that relying largely on the knowledge and experiences of others to provide the answers ultimately does not work. This means that reading countless books, participating in workshops, attending seminars, undertaking spiritual rituals, attendance at religious observances, and being able to regurgitate expounded facts and truths does not guarantee feelings of wellness or inner spiritual growth.

To put it succinctly, talking, reading, and thinking about spirituality do not necessarily result in the attainment of inner peace. These are all mind or intellect activities. They come from the head space, not the heart center. Working with the intellect will generally provide greater knowledge and proficiency of concepts and principles. It is only when the heart center is fully opened and applied to the intellectual knowledge that there can be full integration of the chakras and, from that, attainment of inner peace and enhanced wellness.

This was an ideal time to reflect on a great number of things seen, heard, and experienced in the years of my personal journey and also while helping many others in the course of my work. Often I meet people who have expended a vast amount of time, energy, and money seeking to heal their pain. In many instances a pattern repeats itself. This usually relates to a particular issue an individual seeks to resolve. He or she would do the deep thinking, reflect on the meaning, analyze the issue or situation, and then, when having acquired some level of understanding, would come to the conclusion that the pain had been released.

Surprisingly the same issue would later resurface, and there would be further questioning, searching, and analysis—again with the same result. Very often the individual would be relentless in seeking answers from yet another brilliant teacher, writer, or speaker or from attending another workshop. Ultimately, however, the reality is that no one else has all the answers. You have responsibility for finding the answers that lie within. This is the means by which you gain empowerment and enlightenment.

In order to heal emotional wounds, it is necessary to work with emotions and the heart center, not only the intellect. On a deeper level my friend had been feeling perfectly good about herself and life in general. It was only when she accepted as truth the perception held by someone else that she began to feel distressed. In this regard, my friend's learning was to know that she could trust what she inherently felt within herself. Her innermost feelings were her most reliable barometer! Healing spiritual, emotional, and mental wounds is not a painless process. Anyone who has spent years in therapy attempting to resolve personal and relationship issues revisits countless painful situations in order to achieve understanding and to release the pain from the energy field.

My friends in spirit, my teachers, have shown a straightforward way to have real and lasting healing. It does not have to be protracted. Their teaching is simply that when you bring the energy of love into every situation it changes the dynamics and also yourself in the process. The first place to begin is always with the self. Learning self-love is not widely encouraged in our Western culture. General conditioning is that there is usually more criticism and nonacceptance around personality, appearance, behaviors, and attitudes than there are acceptance and valuing. Self-love begins when there is a change in self-perception from one of continual judgment to one of acceptance. It is not about being narcissistic or hedonistic. There is no room for vanity or pride when coming to a state of self-love. Self-love is accepting fully all aspects of your embodiment.

Energetic Consequences

Your energy field responds to whatever instructions you give it. Think of it as a computer, where everything that happens in your life gets put into the program. How do you wish your program to run? What do you seek from the programming you input? Whatever is placed in the program is returned. Input equals output.

When expressions of self-love, self-worth, and self-acceptance are placed within the energy field, they are returned in multiple ways. The energy field recognizes the vibration of love and thrives on it. The finely tuned grid responds positively. The sensitive thread-like strands regain their strength, flexibility, and balance. When receiving multiple doses of self-love, the grid can be likened to a Christmas tree—it lights up! Simultaneously, the nourishment received from expressions of self-love gradually releases stored emotions, fears, beliefs, and perceptions. The energy of self-love replaces whatever has been released and provides further sustenance to the grid system. The release process relates to issues from this lifetime and all lifetimes. All that you are and ever have been is stored within your energy field.

Love is energy and holds a high vibrational frequency. This frequency has the power to transform and heal whatever is held within your energy field. Coming to a state of total self-acceptance and self-love involves continual awareness of thoughts and behaviors and replacing negative perceptions with the energy of love. It is an ongoing process. Your energy field has the potential to hold infinite light. As you create more nourishment for your energy field, it heals and transforms into an orb of light. It then has the potential to expand even further. This occurs as there is a release of all worldly attachment, and your striving is focused on spiritual enlightenment.

As your energy field fills with self-love and acceptance, there will be changes in your physical experiences. Like attracts like, so you will attract people with similar vibrational frequencies, resulting in new harmonious friendships and relationships. Similarly, you will attract fewer negative issues and experiences into your life. You will find, however, that separation occurs from those whose energies do not align with your new frequencies. Accept this as a natural consequence of the self-healing you are undertaking, and release with love those relationships that do not come from a place of unconditional love.

Creating Self-Love

Coming to a state of self-love releases you from the need for external validation. You know and trust yourself and happily allow your instinctual knowing to guide you. There are positive steps you can take to create a state of self-acceptance and love. As with exercises and suggested strategies in previous chapters, be mindful that change is a process. Be patient with the process and have no expectations as to outcomes. Instead, notice subtle changes and enjoy whatever unfolds.

- Always think and speak positively about yourself. Denigration, self-deprecation, and sarcasm must be eliminated from your vocabulary.

- Monitor thoughts and beliefs you hold about yourself. As soon as a negative thought surfaces, hold it in your mind and then replace it immediately with a loving, nurturing, positive message and image.

- The more this is practiced, the stronger the feelings of self-acceptance and love become. By filling the energy field with supportive and loving thoughts, there is less opportunity for negative perceptions to dominate.

- Continue expressing feelings of self-love, even when it seems a ridiculous exercise and the inner voice of sabotage resists the new tone and language. The barrage of positive words and intentions has energy. They impact the subconscious mind and also affect the whole body, thereby steadily changing the state of the energy field.

- You may discover you hold many beliefs about your unworthiness. Follow the exercise for releasing limiting beliefs described in chapter 14. A great number of these beliefs originate from earlier years and have been reinforced by life experiences.

- Undertake a process of reiteration using only positive intention. This involves more than repeating affirmations countless times. Affirmations have value as they carry energy and intent. However, when they are repeated mindlessly and there are no other changes to thought patterns and beliefs of a negative nature, there is resulting confusion and contradiction in what is intended. Remember, all thoughts, emotions, words, and actions must be in alignment in order to create meaningful and lasting change of a beneficial nature.

- Learn to speak your mind. Ensure that you honor what feels right. Speaking your mind does not mean there is license to speak derogatorily or aggressively. At all times honor the spirit that is in others. Be aware that they too have their truth, even when it conflicts with your truth.

- Undertake activities that add joyfulness and meaning to your life. When doing these, the energy of love will predominate.

- Make it a daily practice to look at yourself directly in the eyes when in front of a mirror and say, "I love me." Hold a steady gaze for some length of time. See the inner beauty you hold. It is a perfectly healthy practice to greet yourself in this manner every morning, especially while still looking unkempt and tousled after a night's sleep. I heartily recommend this strategy for increasing and validating self-love.

- Be aware of the feelings you hold about yourself during this process. Do your emotions match your intentions? It may be of value to spend additional time undertaking the visualization exercise in chapter 15, focusing on bringing compassionate emotions and thoughts into your energy field.

- At every opportunity, ask "How do I feel?" This enables you to connect with the feelings you hold in your heart center. It also assists you to transcend a natural tendency to focus from a mental perspective.

- During this time of transformation, be gentle with yourself. Do things that are nurturing and nourishing. You may choose to purchase a bunch of flowers, go to a show, or enjoy a massage. Do not deny yourself experiences that enhance your sense of self-love.

- Give to others. Make it a daily practice to enrich the life of someone else in some way. It does not have to be for only family or friends. A genuine compliment given to a total stranger does wonders for their morale. Opening the door or offering to help someone when they're obviously experiencing difficulty are other ways to enrich someone else's life. The act of giving unselfishly is enriching. It creates feelings of inner worthiness and warmth.

The journey to seeking and finding self-love varies from person to person, depending on their particular situation. Without self-love, inner peace cannot survive. Be aware that your mind is incredibly powerful, and you have the ability to create a state of mind where peace exists. This peace will continue until such time when an incident occurs or issues arise that trigger unresolved pain. If you have not come to a state of self-acceptance and love, the mind-induced inner peace will be shattered in some way.

The person who assiduously works at releasing feelings of unworthiness and self-hatred and replaces the negative emotions with self-love in time will find their energy field becomes warm and empathic. Those around them will feel this energy vibration as one of genuineness and warmth. When this state is reached, self-trust is also reached. No longer are there doubts about what is right or wrong; no longer is there a need to seek wisdom, answers, or validation from others. When you come to a state of self-love, you know your truth and feel empowered to act in affirming ways.

Signs of Success

How is it possible to determine whether a state of self-love and acceptance has been genuinely integrated and established? A bill of rights for self-lovers is described in *Inner Adventures* and its gist is well worth sharing.[26] As you read through the pertinent points, reflect on whether you have come to this state of self-acceptance and love. If relevant, use this list as a guide for improvement or making changes where you deem necessary.

- As a self-lover, it is perfectly acceptable to be as I choose to be.
- I have the right to think and feel as I choose.
- I am the ultimate judge of my own actions and am responsible for them.
- I have the right and freedom to choose who I love and to allow myself to be loved in return.

---

26. Colin P. Sisson. *Inner Adventures*, Total Press Ltd., 1997.

- I love and respect myself.
- I am able to change, grow, learn, and make mistakes.
- I am responsible for all my actions and thoughts.
- I am able to say "no" without needing the approval of other people.
- My privacy and time alone are important, and I honor that.
- I have the right to ask questions and to expect reasonable answers on matters affecting my life.
- I am trustworthy and expect I will be treated as such.
- If I make a mistake, it is my responsibility to correct it.
- My decisions are my responsibility. It is not necessary to make excuses or justifications.
- It is my responsibility to ensure that I have integrity in all actions without affecting other people adversely.
- I am responsible for solving my problems, for making decisions, and for creating my own happiness.

Inner Radiance

1. *Find a quiet, calm space. Sit comfortably with your feet on the floor and your hands resting in your lap. Close your eyes. Focus your attention on your breath. Bring yourself to a totally relaxed space.*

2. *Bring your consciousness to your energy field. Feel the energies within and around you flowing freely. You may even see your energy grid within this flowing structure.*

3. *Focus your attention on your heart center. It is located midpoint slightly to the right of your physical heart. Feel the energy from your heart center as it flows outward in a vortex. Visualize your heart center opening. Send love from your heart center outward into your energy field. Visualize it as a soft pink color, gradually filling your whole energy field. If you have difficulty doing this, imagine the vortex of energy from your heart center being a fountain, gushing outward and then flowing through your energy field.*

4. *Visualize the energy washing away any negativity, beliefs, and attitudes that are no longer relevant. You may even say a quiet prayer of release if it feels appropriate.*

5. *Feel the changes in your energy field from this additional energy. Feel your energy field expand and strengthen.*

6. *Finally, visualize yourself as a large energy orb, radiating pink energy in all directions. Know that this is the energy of self-love you hold within. It is easily accessible at any time and can be used to strengthen your feelings of self-love and acceptance.*

CHAPTER TWENTY-ONE
Inner Peace

"More calm, more peace, more compassion,
more international feeling
is very good for our health."
—Dalai Lama—

Inner peace is a state of heart and mind. It reflects a certain way of being and seeing the world. The individual who has inner peace does not necessarily have to subscribe to a particular religious or spiritual belief system. Inner peace is a condition that is earned through coming to know yourself and from understanding the world for what it truly is. Inner peace can exist even when chaos and pain predominate in the physical world, as it is not dependent upon or influenced by external conditions.

When there is balance in the mental, emotional, spiritual, and physical levels, inner peace becomes evident. It is created through conscious intent and is the result of hard work and determination. Ironically, inner peace is not necessarily achieved by following a set of prescribed procedures. However, the information, exercises, and strategies shared in this book will provide some assistance in this regard. Most people I know who attain this state attest that the realization of inner peace comes as a surprise.

Below are listed some obvious symptoms of inner peace. As you read each one, check yourself against its relevance to your life. Do you exhibit some or all of the symptoms? To what extent do you exhibit the symptoms? Or do you only occasionally experience any of the symptoms? This is intended as a gentle reminder that changes can be made on a deeper level to allow you to come to a state of peace and harmony in both mind and heart.

Being Joyful

Young children are filled with innocence and joyfulness and respond in this manner to whatever happens. They do not have suitcases of past experiences to load them down each day. They are free, light, optimistic, and effervescent. Past experiences create your perceptions and fears. Learn to overcome these and see them for the limitations of mind they really are. This will free you to be spontaneous and joyful in life.

Thinking and acting joyfully is an invitation to allow your inner child out to play, knowing that the world is a safe place. Allowing the experience of spontaneity to occur for the first time in many years is probably often the most difficult step. After that it becomes easier. It feels liberating and joyful. In doing this you allow the real person, not the one wearing a social mask, to be present.

- Allow yourself to experience the joyfulness of childhood. Find a swing in a park and reexperience the exhilaration of swinging freely.
- Look for the amusing aspects to any situation.
- Learn to laugh, especially at yourself.
- Give gratitude for everything and infuse joyfulness into your thanksgiving.
- Play games with young children. Play games that revitalize you.
- View life as a game, and play the game according to only one rule—to find joy at every opportunity.
- Find joy in relationships and friendships and especially the relationship you have with yourself.

Appreciating Every Moment

This symptom of inner peace appears when you least expect it. When you live totally in the moment and concentrate your attention fully on whatever is happening, you are able to really appreciate whatever is occurring. Whether it is walking through the woods, playing with a young child, preparing a meal for loved ones, or some other mundane chore, it is the act of being fully present and engaged in whatever is happening.

How often do you miss the enjoyment of what is happening at a particular moment because your thoughts are elsewhere? Worries about business, work responsibilities, relationship issues, and family matters are only a few of the common concerns that most people deal with on a regular basis. If there is an issue needing to be resolved, allot time to deal with it, instead of allowing it to intrude into every other aspect of life. Allocating a specific time for thinking and working out strategies, having discussions, and coming to agreements still ensures major issues are resolved in a timely manner. Set aside a specific period of time, say half an hour daily, for this purpose alone. Following a time allocation strategy means that worries do not intrude upon every other waking moment nor interfere with the opportunity for appreciating whatever else is happening.

- Be fully present in all interactions and communications.
- Find the pleasantness (or positive aspects) in every possible situation.
- When in a challenging situation, give gratitude for the experience and learning opportunity.
- Instead of viewing challenges as painful or difficult, look for the positive aspects and then view your learning as enjoyable. This can be achieved when you act as an observer to the situation and understand that the process can become whatever you choose it to be.
- Look for opportunities to laugh.
- Engage your heartfelt emotions when you would normally use your intellect. Feel the difference!

Lacking Desire to Judge or Criticize

Who is your harshest critic? In all probability, it is you. It is not always easy to accept who and what you are, especially as conditioning, media, and advertising usually suggest otherwise. The truth is, you are perfect. The Creator does not judge and accepts you as you are. It is human beings who are critical and judgmental. When you stop viewing the world this way, you will come to see the inherent beauty and goodness in absolutely everything. With the knowing that you are more than your physical body and its limitations, you are then able to recognize your inner beauty. As this occurs, you lose interest in making judgments.

In metaphysical understanding, it is well accepted that when you judge others you are really judging yourself. This means that what is seen in others is also inherent within you to some extent. Making a judgment about someone and determining their value is a limiting exercise. In reality, the human condition is diverse and interesting. Appreciating what another has to offer without making any judgment enables you to experience their depth of character and for that person to feel valued.

- Practice regular acts of kindness toward yourself.
- Practice regular acts of kindness toward others.

- Continually give gratitude for whatever happens.
- As critical thoughts occur, rephrase them into neutral or positive statements.
- Remind yourself, often, that the world is what it is.
- Observe whatever happens without judgment or criticism. This teaches you impartiality and noninvolvement on the emotional and mental levels.

Lacking Interest in Conflict

Whatever happens within is reflected outwardly. When you experience inner conflict, aspects of life will involve conflict with other people. As it is within, so it is without. When there is inner peace, life situations mirror the inner state. Conflict loses its appeal. In situations where there exists a difference of opinion, the person with inner peace will look to achieve a harmonious win-win resolution to problems.

Conflict becomes anathema to the individual who has inner peace. It holds energy that is disruptive and distressing and signifies the polarities still existing in our world. The person who has inner peace knows that everything is One, and, when conflict occurs, it is actually within, which of course there is no need for.

- Seek harmonious solutions to issues and situations as they arise.
- Treat other people as you would like to be treated.
- Whenever a conflict situation occurs, seek out the inner conflict you hold.
- Give thanks when a conflict situation arises as it reveals inner conflict issues that are ready to be healed.
- Practice emotional detachment when conflict arises. This eventually results in reduced intensity in conflicts.
- Practice being peaceful and accepting in your thoughts and emotions.

Being Appreciative

How much of your world do you take for granted? Do you actually notice the numerous beautiful things in your environment? When life becomes filled with stressful demands, there is a tendency to rush busily through each day and to lose sight of what is really important. Remember, energy flows where attention goes, so when your focus is continually on the daily stresses, they define your experience of life.

Once a state of inner peace is attained, you will find a busy life is only one small layer within everything else that exists. With inner peace you see and know the consciousness of others in your community; you feel their strivings and understand the perfection of everything. The world is in perfect working order. Mother Nature provides an abundance that is accessible to all. When you have this awareness, the feelings of overwhelming appreciation will well up from within. These are the emotions of gratitude and of feeling blessed.

- Consciously practice giving gratitude for all you have.
- Pay attention to the inherent beauty in your environment.
- Appreciate other people.
- Appreciate your special gifts and talents.
- Value your physical body. Be appreciative of all that it does for you.
- Begin each day joyfully.
- Always go to bed in a calm state.

Feeling Connected

As an adult, it is easy to view others with mistrust and as being different. A perceived state of separation from all others is reinforced by normal life experiences. You are brought up to believe that the world is not a safe place, that your neighbors are not to be trusted, and to judge people by their religion, color, or ethnic background. Is it any wonder that it is common to view anything that is unfamiliar with suspicion?

In your spiritual seeking you will recognize the erroneousness of feeling suspicion and separation. You will recognize that all is One. The essence of the Divine Source is within you, and it is this that connects you to the One. Energetically it can be expressed differently. As everything is energy, there can be no separation for there is never empty space anywhere in the great cosmic universe. The energy web of life connects everything.

When experiencing this particular symptom of inner peace, there can be no judgment or rejection of whatever occurs. The homeless person, the lottery winner, and the drought-stricken earth are all part of the One. Whatever they feel, the person with inner peace feels. There is no distinction. Feelings of connectedness occur when there is a recognition of others as being within the One and doing so with compassion and love in your heart center.

- Suspend judgment and criticism whenever the tendency surfaces. Instead, replace those thoughts with either neutral or positive statements.
- Learn to value the similarities in people.
- Appreciate the differences.
- Open your mind to seeing issues and situations from differing perspectives.
- Spend time in nature. Marvel at its stunning beauty. Feel yourself enveloped by and connected with its energies.

Living from the Heart Center

In order to know universal unconditional love, it has to be experienced within as well as extended to others. However, societal conditioning has us believe it is normal to hate people, issues, and situations. Hatred is not a natural state. You were not born to hatred; you were trained into it! Hatred can be untrained. This occurs when you make a conscious decision to let go of hatred and learn to love without judgment. Learning to love entails letting go of many beliefs and emotions. Yet the more it is practiced, the easier it becomes until such time it assumes a natural state.

Living from the heart center involves bringing compassion, tolerance, acceptance, and empathy to every situation. It means relegating the intellect to the back seat and allowing feeling to predominate in all life situations.

- Learn to recognize and value the special unique qualities in every person.
- Accept yourself and other people as they are.
- Let go of any resentment and anger you hold.
- Become familiar and comfortable with your feelings. Many people intellectualize how they feel. There is a significant difference!
- Practice extending compassion instead of criticism.

Each of these symptoms of inner peace reflects a profound wisdom regarding how life can be lived with purpose, love, and trust. Some of the spiritual truths and principles discussed in this chapter will be expanded in greater detail in the following chapters. Making time to concentrate energy and intent on achieving any or all of the symptoms is the first step toward achieving inner harmony and peace. Being consistently constructive and positive in thoughts and emotions eventually results in greater acceptance of what is. There will be less judgment and fear and more trust that well-being and safety are a birthright.

On a global level, the majority of humanity desires world peace. There are many organizations and peace movements worldwide dedicated to achieving international peace and cooperation. However, I remember clearly the words from my friends in spirit regarding the achievement of world peace. These words were shared around the time of the attack on the World Trade Center in New York. My friends were observing what had occurred, our human responses and emotions, and simply stated, "How can there be world peace when there is no peace within the hearts of humanity?"

Often these words resurface in my mind, and I wonder whether globally we are truly any closer to having peace in our hearts. World peace can never be a reality until the time when the majority of the world's population achieves that calm state of inner peace. All the endeavors toward world peace will not occur while emotions of mistrust, anger, and fear continue to fester within and between nations.

It is your responsibility to focus intention and energy inward to find that inner calm place. When you find that state, everything changes. Your perceptions of the world and yourself undergo a dramatic shift. Nothing changes, yet everything changes. In changing yourself, there is actually a change in the world. Surprisingly, once that inner peace is found, anger dissipates. Instead there is acceptance with compassion. There is no longer the need to be zealous in creating change or trying to convince people of your convictions because you accept that each human being is on an individual journey and is doing the very best they can, given life circumstances.

Being in a state of inner peace involves releasing attitudes and beliefs that are no longer valid, thereby enabling your energy field to blossom. A constant diet of gentleness, gratitude, acceptance, compassion, and love further strengthen the energy field. In this invigorated state, the energy field is no longer readily susceptible to negativity. As the energy field strengthens, there are significant changes within the emotional, mental, and physical levels. The energy field clears toxins and blocked energies, thereby increasing its light frequency. In time, the results become evident in the physical body as conditions heal.

CHAPTER TWENTY-TWO
Loving
Forgiveness

"Life will bring you pain all by itself.
Your responsibility is to create joy."
—Milton Erickson, M.D.—

Love heals all things. This is true, both literally and figuratively. When working with the intention of releasing old pain and infusing your body with the energy of love, beneficial changes occur on every level. This is because the vibration of love is so strong that it is capable of healing the blockages sitting in the energy grid and any other damage that has been created over the years. Even though you may not be able to see the healing that takes place, on a subtle level you begin to feel the benefits within a relatively short period of time. You will experience heightened awareness within and in external reality. Mentally and emotionally you will feel lighter, calmer, and clearer. Physical changes gradually become evident as you honor your body and ensure that it too receives only premium quality nourishment. When you come to a state of self-love, you have no choice but to value your physical body and to ensure that, like a car, it is maintained at an optimal level.

Conditional Love

Earlier I wrote about unconditional love. In order to understand what this means, it is necessary to understand the difference between conditional, or emotional, and unconditional love. It is easy to confuse the two. Emotional love is the love you have for your significant partner, children, parents, and so on. You grow up accepting emotional love from your family. Generally, it is conditional and based on assumptions of what love actually means. How often do you hear, "If he/she really loved me then . . ." Or "Be a good boy/girl and . . ." From an early age you learn that there are terms and conditions on the love that is given by family and friends. This, in turn, is accepted as being normal, and the same patterning continues as you grow into adulthood and into interactions you have with loved ones.

Often the conditions are subtle and ingrained, and you do not realize they have been imposed. Examples of this are abundantly evident and include:

- expecting someone to change their nature because they love you;

- rewarding someone with a special treat because they have done as you wished;

- doing something for a loved one with the underlying hope that you will get what is really desired; and

- blaming someone because they have hurt you in some way.

There is no denying that reactions and responses occur according to upbringing, which shapes your perception of what love means.

Emotional love results in pain. The reason for this is that there are conditions, expectations, and judgments (often implicit and mutually agreed upon) imposed in meaningful relationships. One result is that it is common for people to end up feeling disappointed, vulnerable, disillusioned, and wary about loving too much. If I were to have a dollar for every client I have seen that has been hurt in love, who has become cynical and is fearful of feeling love again, I would indeed be a wealthy woman!

Unconditional Love

A critical step to achieving peace of mind and general well-being involves coming to a state of unconditional love. This is the love that is written about in the Scriptures. It is what the enlightened masters and gurus refer to in their teachings. Buddha, Krishna, Jesus, Mohamed, and others of infinite wisdom and love have shown how to live a truly worthy life. Their purpose in coming to earth was to achieve this state of being, to live exemplary lives, and to teach that it is possible for us to come to know this love.

Unconditional love is not bound by conditions or expectations. It is universal energy, readily available and given freely. The difference between emotional love and unconditional love is that emotions have attachment whereas unconditional love has none. Unconditional love is a state that all people have the capacity to attain. In order to do so, it means letting go of emotional attachment and expectations.

Attaining a state of unconditional love literally involves unlearning old ways of thinking and feeling. It means discarding long-held perceptions about who you are and the limitations that have been set in place. When in a state of unconditional love, you see the inner beauty and accept the perfection in everything. Even the perceived imperfections are perfect!

One of the first and most critical steps in undertaking self-healing is to come to a state of self-love. Everything changes as a result of undergoing this transformational process. It becomes easier to implement a healthy diet regime and other practical healing strategies because now the emphasis is on truly knowing and valuing the self. The inner voice of sabotage no longer plays a predominant role in creating mayhem or distracting you to behave in ways that are detrimental to well-being. Self-love comes from the heart. The mind has no influence on it. In fact, much of the self-sabotage that is customary in daily life comes from the ego consciousness or mind. When the heart center is fully open and the energy of love flows freely, the mind can be utilized for its rightful purpose, which is expanded thinking and processing.

Opening your heart to the energy of love may initially feel uncomfortable and threatening. The reason for this is that life experiences often result in emotional scarring, leading to a lack of trust in relationships. Often a wall is literally placed around the heart in order to prevent further hurt. Though this wall may be invisible, it is real nevertheless. The wall consists of the emotion that has been expended in its construction. It sits over and well into the fourth chakra, which is the heart chakra or heart center.

As the journey into self-love is undertaken, the heart chakra begins to open up as old emotional wounds are healed. The more the heart center is imbued with the energy of love, the further it will open and the higher its vibration will become. Compassion and the energy of unconditional love radiate outward and become a strong palpable force that is instantly recognized and felt by other people.

Why Forgive?

Strategies for creating the energy of self-love have been clearly described in a previous chapter. In undertaking this exciting inner transformation, it is important to include the aspect of forgiveness in the healing process. Many of the Scriptures teach the need for forgiveness so that healing can occur. Coming to a state of self-love means accepting totally who you are and what you have done. There can be no judgment or regret over past events.

You are the sum total of all your experiences. Many of those experiences may have been enjoyable, others far from enjoyable and maybe even downright embarrassing and shameful. However, all those experiences in which you behaved badly or inappropriately are the best teachers. It is from mistakes that the most profound learning occurs. It is what you do with what has been learned from those mistakes that is important. Viewing transgressions as an opportunity to learn and grow affords the opportunity to place previous wrongdoings into an entirely new and healthy perspective.

This is why forgiveness is so relevant to the healing process. Hanging onto past mistakes and behaviors with feelings of guilt involves self-judgment and criticism. It also involves placing energy into the past, rather than living fully in the moment. Regrets and recriminations have no place in the heart center. There are many ways of undergoing the process of forgiveness. It is as necessary to forgive yourself as it is to forgive those whom you feel have inflicted hurt.

Self-Forgiveness

Self-forgiveness occurs when you stop concentrating on past incidents and accept what has happened without recrimination or judgment. It enables the release of blocked energy around old emotional wounds. When you recognize the need to forgive someone, this is an indication that self-forgiveness is also needed. As with all healing, this is a gradual process. Accept it as a journey of self-discovery and exploration. If you are not sure where to begin or how to proceed, the following may be helpful.

- Whenever a memory surfaces that is a reminder of past mistakes and where there is still an element of judgment, it is an appropriate time to reflect on what happened.

- During that reflection, consciously communicate to yourself that you forgive yourself. This forgiveness may be for pain you have self-inflicted or may have inflicted on someone else.

- If it involves someone else, silently ask his or her forgiveness after you have sincerely forgiven yourself.

- This process carries energy and intent, and when forgiveness comes from the heart (and not mind), it releases the pain of that memory.

- Prayer is another highly effective means of working with forgiveness. In your prayers, forgive yourself as well as others.

- Writing is another efficient means of releasing past pain and dealing with forgiveness issues. One strategy is to write down everything relating to a specific person or issue and at the end express complete forgiveness. When this is done, there is no need to reread what has been written. You may wish to burn the paper as this releases the energy and signifies completion.

- When you are calm ask yourself four questions:
  1. When did this issue really begin?
  2. Why did this happen?
  3. What have I learned from this?
  4. How can I apply this learning to future situations?

Your answers will reveal significant information about the extent of the emotional and mental wounds you hold. Use the suggested strategies and visualizations contained in this book to assist you further with their release.

Forgiving Others

Saying "I forgive you" is not easy for most people. Usually when there are emotional issues, past resentments, and other symptoms of pain in relationships, honest and open communication is affected. Forgiveness works when it comes from the heart center. It has to be genuine. I have learned a strategy that can be applied at any time and that peels back the layers of pain every time it is practiced.

Communicating energetically with the person involved is a straightforward process and is extremely powerful. This process is internal and is outlined below. The intention creates the same outcome as if you had addressed them personally. By this I mean that it changes your feelings about the situation and the person.

- Find a quiet place and calm your mind before following this process.

- Call the person energetically by name three times. Say, "I call in (name)."

- As you do this, you will feel their essence come to you.

- Talk to that person as if he or she were there in person. Whatever is expressed relates specifically to the issues and emotions that exist between you.

- During the conversation, state explicitly that you have forgiven both yourself and them.

- Conclude your conversation with a statement expressing loving wishes toward them.

- This process may take some time and is incredibly powerful in its healing. The intention is always to honor the other person, to honor your feelings, and to clear the issue or emotion involved. When this process is undertaken in the spirit of love, with no negative emotions involved, the release experienced can be cathartic.

There may be times when the forgiveness process requires numerous attempts, each of them genuine and heartfelt. This is because often there are more issues involved than are readily recognized, or it may be that on a subtle level you are willing to forgive only so much and not the whole gamut. Be patient with yourself and the process if you find yourself caught in a pattern of repeating the forgiveness ceremony. To speed the process, you may choose to ask yourself the four questions listed under Self-Forgiveness. The answers may provide greater insight into the depth and extent of the emotional wounds you hold.

listed under Self-Forgiveness. The answers may provide greater insight into the depth and extent of the emotional wounds you hold.

When you undertake this energetic process of forgiveness, you may find there is no need to express your forgiveness verbally to the person concerned. The emotional issues will dissipate as you acquire understanding and acceptance of what has happened, thereby reducing or even eliminating the need for verbal expression.

Energy Benefits

The magic contained within this process of acquiring self-love and forgiveness is priceless. As you come to this state, you suspend judgment and negativity. Energy becomes focused on the positive aspects, and the vibration of love strengthens. When you feel the Divine essence of love and beauty within, you also come to recognize it in everything else. The negativity and hatred perceived in others and also felt toward them are merely a reflection of where you started. As the negative energies within dissipate, you view the world differently, and, best of all, you will feel lighter and calmer on all levels.

Whenever acts of forgiveness are undertaken, there is a release of negativity from within the energy field. Loving, nurturing energy then replaces the blockage caused by the stored negativity. A friend doing healing work recently described it clearly. She saw a dark mass leaving the energy field, and immediately the energy grid was restored to its natural structural form. She also commented that, as this happened, the grid became clear with light emanating from it.

When there is self-love, the energy of unconditional love emanates from within. This is soul food to your energy field. As you concentrate your efforts to work from the heart center, the energy field gains in strength and health. It is as though the energy field literally sloughs off the detritus of negativity, emotional and mental pain, and old stagnant energies. It becomes alive and vibrant. The more you work with the energy of love, the healthier your body becomes. Positive energy and intent are to your body what chemical-free fertilizer is to soil. The more goodness and positive energies you radiate, the richer your harvest will be!

I would like to share the words of a great teacher: "Any act against Love is an act against good health. Any time a man acts against the principle of Love, he creates short circuits in his energy network. Love is life. Actions against Love are actions against life. This is true for the individual, for a family, for a nation, and for all humanity. Violation of the Love principle creates various disturbances, not only within our emotional nature but also within our mental nature and within our social and international life. Free circulation of the Love principle is the answer to most of our health problems."[27]

Compassionate Forgiveness

The suggestions in this chapter for undertaking forgiveness can be supported by visualization. When doing this visualization, the intention is to connect with the heart center, thereby strengthening the forgiveness process.

- *Find a quiet, calm space. Sit comfortably with your feet flat on the floor and your hands resting in your lap. Focus on your breath. Breathe deeply and slowly. Feel the tension leaving your body and your mind become calm.*

- *When you find yourself in a relaxed state where outside thoughts have faded, bring to your consciousness a forgiveness issue you are choosing to release. It would be preferable if you have already undertaken some of the steps described earlier in this chapter.*

- *Visualize this forgiveness issue as being encapsulated within a large dark mass that is sitting within your energy field. You feel its weight as it rests in one of your chakras—usually in the first three chakras and sometimes in the heart center.*

- *Now feel your heart center expand and open wide. Do this by focusing your intention on the heart chakra. Feel it spinning in a vortex and gradually expanding. Visualize it as spilling outward. You may even see it as a color—possibly green, pink, or gold.*

---

27. Torkom Saraydarian. *New Dimensions in Healing*, T.S.G. Publishing Foundation, Inc.,1992.

- Feel the energy moving from your heart center and into your whole energy field. As you do this, you will feel sensations of warmth or tingling within your physical body.

- Now move the energy to the area where your forgiveness issue sits. Gently feel the energy from your heart center push out the dark mass. You may find some initial resistance. If so, concentrate your thoughts on sending love and healing while continuing to feel the heart center pushing gently to release the blockage.

- As the forgiveness issue releases, you will feel a sensation of something being pulled out of your energy field. This will result in a feeling of lightness in the area.

- Maintain your focus on the area of the blockage release. What do you see? Are you able to see the energy grid whole and filled with light? When ready, gradually bring your focus back to your breathing and finally, bring your attention back to the room.

CHAPTER TWENTY-THREE
Soul Essence

"The smarter a person is,
the more they need Great Spirit
to protect them
from thinking they know it all.
Only Great Spirit knows all!"
—Son of White Cloud—

As you read this book and begin implementing changes in relevant areas, you will begin to notice steady improvement on all levels. Some of the changes may initially be subtle. In time there will be significant progress in both well-being and health, provided you continue with the suggestions and exercises. Be patient with the process. All that I share and advocate requires time and commitment for improvement to become apparent.

When something is awry in life, it is usual to identify an obvious area of deficit needing attention or change. This approach, while helpful, has limitations, as the conscious mind is not always the most reliable arbiter of inner needs. My approach to wellness and self-healing involves the balanced integration of the physical, mental, emotional, and spiritual levels. Through a process of steadily letting go of preconceptions and expectations and allowing your soul to be the guide as to what is in your best interest, healing occurs on a deeper level. Eventually this produces greater balance in practically every area of life.

The changes initially implemented take effect in the outer layers of your energy field before gradually manifesting on the physical level. I have observed this process in many instances as clients report increased feelings of well-being in their emotions and mental outlook long before there are indications of healing occurring in the physical body. It has also been my experience that for healing to be lasting, it is vital to incorporate the suggested spiritual practices into daily life. Spiritual practice enhances healing of the energy field. The positive energy you direct toward yourself, others, and the planet will return to you magnified.

In addition to the practical suggestions shared in this book, there are other principles that, when applied, enhance the healing process and increase well-being. Even when there is little or no indication of any physical illness or condition existing, daily stresses accumulate that gradually have a debilitating impact on the quality of life. The principles shared in this and the following chapters are subtle yet nonetheless equally powerful when implemented with the intention of creating a life of wellness, abundance, and meaning.

Living in the Moment

The practice of living in the moment is one that cannot be stressed too highly. Being in the moment is self-explanatory. It literally means living in the present no matter whatever else has ever occurred or will possibly eventuate. Learning to live in the moment is challenging. Conditioning has trained most people to focus energy on imagining the possibility of various scenarios occurring in daily life and then how best to deal with them. These are distractions and can be eliminated.

The antitheses of living in the moment are worry and regret. Stress results from worry-induced thinking. Worry is a process of mind activity comprising mainly endless and inane mind chatter. It is a projection into future possibilities based on past perceptions, experiences, and fears. Worry indicates a belief that things always remain the same or that because something has happened it will happen again. Wrong! When this belief is held, you actually create more of the same because your reality originates from the thoughts you hold.

All worries (fears) can eventually become an instrument for learning. When there is recognition that worry is intangible, it can then be released because it has no basis in substance. Its intangibility resides in the mind, and, when it is replaced with calmness and acceptance, it loses its grip on reality. Daily meditation and quiet time for giving gratitude assist in releasing relentless mind chatter.

Regret occurs when energy is directed to past events, people, and issues. Most people express regret over something said, done, or maybe not done. The past is the past and cannot be undone. However, what you choose to learn from it and how you behave as a consequence are potent signs that the lesson has been meaningful. This is where self-forgiveness becomes critical to healing old wounds and regrets.

Holding on to memories of past times or to hanker nostalgically for a different time or memory is another means of avoiding the present moment. A man I met preferred to listen to music from the sixties and seventies. His conversation continually reminisced on the wonderful times he had experienced in that era. Obviously that era contained many warm memories. However, he appeared to be stuck emotionally. He had not let go of the past and therefore was unable to see the beauty and exciting possibilities in his present life.

Living in the moment does not mean jeopardizing or ignoring goal setting and planning around major life commitments and decisions. There is great value in goal setting and being organized, whether in relation to career direction or organizing major projects. Allocate appropriate time to the organization and planning and then follow the tasks in a timely manner, dealing with whatever demands attention as it arises. Simultaneously, by having the forward planning in place, it is possible to prevent likely glitches.

Applying energy and attention to what needs to be done at the appropriate time minimizes the potential for worry and agitation in any life situation. Similarly, with adequate forward planning, there is still the possibility of making relevant changes as necessary depending on whatever is happening in the moment. Goal setting and forward planning do not mean inflexibility. Instead, they can be viewed as a means of enhancing life choices while minimizing worry or stress.

Being fully present in awareness is the key to living in the moment. It means having full consciousness of whatever is occurring. Making the decision to be fully present is the first step toward achieving the joy of living in the now. Sometimes it can be more alluring to daydream or to imagine exotic events, as they offer an escape from the perceived dreariness of daily life. Living in the moment forces you to give full attention to whatever is happening. When this occurs, it is easy to see the beauty in everything and to marvel at the abundance at your disposal.

My friends in spirit have reiterated numerous times the importance of living in the present moment. They express it very succinctly: "Now is all you have." It is the only moment that exists and is all the more precious because of its uniqueness. If living in the moment is a new experience you may wish to adopt the following strategies.

- Begin by making simple changes to your thinking. Every time you find yourself focusing energy in the past, stop your train of thought and consciously concentrate on whatever is happening in the present moment.

- When you worry about a future possibility, do the same. Bring your attention to the present moment.

- Set a goal to live fully in the moment for an hour daily. Allow no thoughts of the past or future to intrude during this allocated time.

- While in the moment, feel what is happening. Look at its beauty. Give gratitude for the special magic that is occurring. Feel yourself relaxing, as there is nothing to worry about and nothing to do but just be in the present moment.

- Increase your time allocation for being in the moment to half a day at a time, then a full day, a week, and so on. When you do this, recognize that there may be thoughts intruding that demand your attention.

- Acknowledge those thoughts and affirm silently that they will be dealt with at a time when you are choosing to not live in the moment. Most likely, when you are ready to deal with those intrusive thoughts, you will realize they are not necessarily relevant or important.

In time you will give your attention to those things that require your focus only when it is absolutely appropriate. You will discover there will not be any preconceived perceptions and fears associated with them, as there would have been had you allowed yourself to dwell upon them needlessly.

Acceptance

How often do you find yourself saying, "If only I had done . . ." or "Why did he or she behave as they did?" or "It isn't right; it should be this way . . ." Whatever decisions or actions are taken, it is always easier, upon reflection, to see another more appropriate response. The desire for the perfect response, behavior, and outcome involves judgment and nonacceptance of what has transpired. Taken to an extreme it can become increasingly easy to always find fault and to never be satisfied with situations or people.

Coming to accept that things are what they are is another simple spiritual awareness that assists healing and inner growth. Upon attaining a state of self-love and self-acceptance, it is basically a matter of extending those states to everything else. This means there is no room for judgment, criticism, or negativity in perception, thought, or action. Whether a glass is half full or half empty becomes irrelevant. It has no meaning attached to it and is what it is.

It is a natural inclination to be critical with the imperfections seen every day in our world. Defining people and things as good or bad and right or wrong is a customary behavior. Limitations and faults in others are quickly discerned. All these traits are a reflection of what is seen within yourself, as everything and everyone is your mirror! When you accept what is, then there is no right or wrong, no imperfection, and no room for judgment or negativity.

- Learn to suspend judgment; instead, accept that someone else behaves in ways that are meaningful to him or her.
- Accept that your choices and decisions are not necessarily appropriate for other people, as theirs may not be of your choosing.
- Accept that people do the very best with whatever means they have at their disposal.
- Extend compassion to others. This involves honoring other peoples' awareness and life journey. Literally, it means accepting them as they are and not as you would like them to be.
- Stop questioning and analyzing everything that happens, as this is another form of resistance. When you accept whatever happens, understanding will occur in a timely manner. This understanding is also likely to be of a deeper nature, rather than the superficial understanding that is gained through logical reasoning.
- Know that all things will pass. Today's trauma will become a memory. Tomorrow's exciting event will also become a memory. Accept whatever is happening right at this very moment.
- Instead of becoming angry at perceived injustices or political ideologies, accept that other people also have the right to their experiences and life choices.

When you experience a health-related condition, accept it as being part of your life experience. Ill health occurs for a reason. Accepting what has happened is critical to undertaking the healing process. A client experienced a number of health conditions that forced his early retirement. His healing has been slow as he refuses to accept his ill health. Acknowledging and accepting the conditions and the constraints they place will eventually enable his body to begin healing. Even creating the thought "I used to have diabetes" or whatever the condition may be accepts and honors what has occurred. Accept what has happened and then commence the process of changing beliefs, perceptions, and energy around the condition or situation.

Nonattachment

Nonattachment involves having no attachment or expectation in relation to people, issues, beliefs, and situations. This state of being is generally difficult to understand and achieve in any spiritual journey. General conditioning teaches the exact opposite. From the time of birth, you are imbued with beliefs regarding the importance of caring for others. Somehow the idea is planted that you are responsible for and involved in whatever happens to other people. From this it becomes acceptable to demonstrate caring (and attachment) through emotions.

In truth, you are only responsible for how you live your life. At the soul level, you know very well and understand what is appropriate and necessary for your personal growth and awareness. What other people choose to do and how they live is their responsibility. At all times trust that each person knows what is the best course of action for him or her.

It is often easy to see the potential for disaster in decisions people make, yet these very disasters usually provide an opportunity for real growth. It is not for you to judge or determine what is the wisest course of action for anyone else. Sometimes standing back and observing with compassion and nonattachment can be difficult, especially when there is shared emotional connection or fondness. A dear friend became romantically involved with a man. In almost no time all his business affairs were placed in her name, and he lied about his financial and business matters. Eventually the dishonesty and lies surfaced, and she faced bankruptcy as a consequence of his actions. Nowadays she gives thanks for that experience, as it has been a gift in many ways. She has unearthed inner strength and discovered a talent for dealing with debt collectors and financial institutions as well as an ability to negotiate with confidence and clarity. In addition, she has no attachment to the money lost nor does she view the relationship as anything but a positive learning experience.

Nonattachment is an essential state to be in when working with clients. I cannot become emotionally involved in their welfare or have any expectations around their healing process. Rather, it is important to give 100 percent professionally to each client while knowing how they respond is an individual matter. When working with clients who have a serious illness, it is their choice, at the soul level, as to whether they remain or transition. Having attachment would involve a myriad of emotions, including self-recrimination, anger, and fear if things did not turn out in a manner I would have wished. It is not for me to know or presume to know what is for another's highest good.

Nonattachment is evident when you accept that every person has the ability to deal with any life situation that arises, no matter how tough it may be. In viewing life challenges in this manner, it becomes easier to deal with whatever occurs, especially when having no expectations in regard to outcomes. Having no attachment or expectations allows you to be fully in the moment, have greater peace of mind, and to also explore creatively all possible options.

Nonattachment is a way of being, and there are several strategies that can be employed in practicing this. Be mindful that while practicing nonattachment, you will most likely be learning the state of acceptance. The two seem to go hand in hand.

- One particularly effective way of achieving nonattachment is to practice being a witness to incidents. This includes events that involve the self as well as others. As an observer, there is no emotional attachment, subjective analysis, or expectation. There are merely observational insights, and it then becomes a matter of gleaning some understanding and awareness of the underlying beliefs and issues. With this awareness in place, you are in a better position to act appropriately.

- Whenever a situation or issue arises, ask a simple question: "Who owns the problem?" If, after careful scrutiny and reflection, the issue or emotion is yours, then it is your responsibility. However, if the issue belongs to someone else, it becomes his or her obligation to resolve. It is important to trust that other people have the ability to problem solve their particular situations or issues. These provide a learning opportunity and offer a means of growth in awareness and understanding. If you believe it is your duty to deal with all problems or issues that you see, then you are literally depriving other people of critical learning opportunities.

- When a situation arises involving someone else, stop before you speak and act in response. Question your motives. Focus on your emotional reaction. Assess what would be gained by your input and involvement. By all means become a participant if that is your choosing. However, by taking time to question, you allow yourself to become emotionally uninvolved (or in a state of nonattachment).

- Nonattachment also applies to material possessions and external reality. Assess your level of attachment to the material possessions you own and to all other external factors. Which ones can you live without? How would you feel if you were deprived of all your important mementos and possessions? Your reaction to these questions reveals the level of attachment you have.

By the way, nonattachment does not mean lack of compassion. In fact, the opposite is true. In a state of nonattachment, you are best able to extend tolerance, compassion, and love. This is because nonattachment has no conditions. When you are in this state, you are accepting of whatever is and know that each person is a powerful being with capabilities they are still in the process of discovering.

Letting Go

Letting go is aligned with the states of acceptance and nonattachment. It involves trusting that whatever happens is perfect, even when no effort is expended to ensure specific outcomes. There is a higher force than your conscious mind that is perfectly capable of ensuring life choices and directions are in alignment with your soul's intent.

The opposite of this state is the desire and determination to be in control. Often I hear people say it is important to them to be in control of their life, finances, or other people. Have you ever had the experience of believing in a certain life path and had the determination to pursue relevant goals? A client shared this story. No matter how hard he tried, success was elusive. His commitment and endeavors would invariably fail, and he would then be left asking, "Why?" Eventually he heard the statement, "Let go, let God." Fortuitously he interpreted this to mean that it was time to take his hands off the steering wheel and allow a higher source to provide guidance.

Happily he relinquished control, and amazing changes began happening in positive and surprising ways. It was not long, however, before habit resurfaced, and slowly he began to reassert his dominance of the steering wheel. Again, blocked walls appeared at every turn. It seemed that whenever he attempted to take control he was quickly reminded of his ineptness! Needless to say, the process occurred several times until he finally acquiesced and handed control over to a higher source. One consequence of this is that he now has greater uncertainty in his life, as changes occur with regular monotony. Life has become more of an adventure with many diverse experiences occurring that he could never have dreamt of creating. In letting go of the need to control he has learned to trust his intuition implicitly.

In our culture, managing tasks and people readily becomes a way of life. It requires a great deal of energy and consumes an inordinate amount of time in order to ensure that everything happens according to planned outcomes. Needless to say, living like this for any period of time creates additional stress within the body, even if it is not immediately apparent. Worry and stress are linked to adverse health conditions, including heart disease, high blood pressure, and gastric disorders.

Letting go literally means handing over the reins to a higher source. This involves trust and acceptance that whatever occurs is for the highest good. It does not necessarily involve abrogation of responsibilities or the foregoing of decision-making in daily issues. So, how is it possible to begin the process of letting go?

- Whenever you have the urge to take control or manage something or someone, stop, step back, and allow events to unfold in their own way.

- When the urge to take charge is strong, question the reason for this. Assess how you would feel if you were not in charge. Explore the emotions and beliefs you hold around the need to be in control. The underlying emotion is likely to be a deep-seated fear. Once you have an understanding of the fear, it loses its power, especially once the process of releasing the baseless fear is underway.

- Listen to the guidance of your inner voice, or intuition. This will guide you in unexpected ways, enabling you to experience life as a spiritual being and not necessarily controlled by fears and conscious resistance. The more you learn to trust your inner voice, the easier life becomes.

- Allow situations and issues to unfold without always having to be in control. You will observe that events have a natural and easy way of unfolding, and, consequently, stress levels will be reduced considerably.

- Trust you will always be looked after. Situations generally work out in unexpected and surprising ways that are usually beneficial.

Energy Expansion

The principles of living in the moment, having acceptance, living with nonattachment, and letting go have been explored briefly. Learning and experiencing each of these principles is a complex process. When undertaking a spiritual journey, you will attract each of these in their many forms as opportunities for further learning. Having intellectual knowledge of the principles does not necessarily constitute internalized learning. When you absorb and know them intimately within the heart center, living them becomes easy.

The benefits of integrating these principles into daily life become evident in your energy field. Immediately there is relief on the physical, mental, and emotional levels, as the principles themselves support a stress-free life. The energy of worry, regret, and countless other emotions no longer impinge upon your consciousness. The mind is freed from relentless chatter, and stored clutter is released. The physical body is no longer affected by constant adrenaline surges, which are a common fight-or-flight response triggered by emotional and mental reactions.

Without the continual input of emotions and thoughts that are damaging to the energy field, the opportunity exists for it to be stabilized and balanced. However, nothing in the universe is ever static. Even when the energy field is in a state of homeostasis, it continues to expand. The energy of the spiritual principles continually applied in everyday situations is added to the existing structure. Imagine the energy grid as a core, whole within itself. This is the structure that you continually strive to maintain in good health. Now imagine this core as being balanced and receiving additional nourishment on a continuous basis. The additional nourishment can only add to what is already in existence. The core, already healed and whole, can only expand.

The core is filled with light energy as healing releases emotional blockages, beliefs, and old wounds. Like attracts like, so the core attracts additional light. As the spiritual principles are applied from the heart center, these flow outward to impact on everything and everyone else. In addition, like a boomerang, they return to the energy field where they are then stored. The more these spiritual principles are applied in everyday situations, the greater the rewards in terms of creating an energy grid that is strong, vital, and filled with light.

CHAPTER TWENTY-FOUR
Energy and Positive Living

"We must be the change we wish to see in the world."
—Mahatma Gandhi—

Right Living

The Scriptures and other holy books expound the virtues of right living. This concept covers a multitude of positive attributes and behaviors, all of which add considerably to the quality of life. Generally, right living encompasses all the attributes that nourish the soul. Being truthful, thinking positively, living compassionately, being of service, finding joy and peace, having integrity, and being authentic are some of the qualities that imbue the energy field with healing and expansion.

Here the term "right" is not used as meaning the opposite of wrong but more as a characteristic that is in alignment with the purpose of the soul. "Right" is a context that is easily identifiable and encompasses broader socially acceptable behaviors and attitudes. It is not a signifier of judgment nor used as a basis for comparison.

Earlier it was mentioned that whatever is given out is also received or returned. As an example, when feelings of anger and hostility are expressed, they not only strike the object of your emotions but also rebound like a boomerang and land back in your energy field. In other words, there is a double-whammy effect whenever any emotion is expressed. The intended recipient either receives positive or negative emotional energy, which impacts his or her energy field. The sender receives the same energy with magnified impact. Logically it makes sense to always ensure that only compassionate thoughts and emotions are transmitted.

When the intention is focused on having compassion, helping other people, being loving in thoughts and actions, and honoring all of creation, the energy field undergoes healing. The impact of spiritual practice and right living gradually replaces the blocked energy stored within the energy field, resulting in increased well-being and vitality. The greater the consistency of right living, the stronger the energy field becomes. The more you strive to ensure harmony in all endeavors, the greater the rewards.

As the energy field is healed, emotional distortions and blockages are replaced with light energy. This light is universal unconditional love. The more right living is practiced, the more the energy field is filled with light energy. This is the process of enlightenment—literally meaning to be filled with light. I remember asking my friends in spirit how much light the body could hold and was told the amount is infinite.

Other right living qualities include being joyful, having purpose, being gentle, practicing harmlessness, and purity of thought. Joyfulness involves experiencing delight in everything. I have noticed that highly evolved beings exhibit a simplicity of joyfulness. They find an almost childlike delight in all things. They see the beauty in nature and are in awe and appreciative of the many beautiful and natural wonders of life. Laughter and smiling come naturally and spontaneously.

Having purpose does not necessarily mean achieving great worldly success and recognition. It means possessing inner knowing of what the soul's purpose is in its incarnation. This may simply be to learn love and to live life to the very best of your ability. It may involve contributing meaningfully and creatively to your community. Or it may be to learn the qualities of acceptance and forgiveness. The purpose is then integrated into all other aspects of daily life, thereby engendering a sense of direction and inner completeness.

Gentleness is probably anathema to the conditioning received by most people in the Western world. Societal mores value and externalize violence and cruelty. These are endemic in movies, television, and video games and reflect the acts of barbarism inflicted upon our brothers and sisters within society and also upon those of other cultures. When you speak, think, and act with gentleness, you are emitting an energy that is conducive to healing the energy field. Violence and cruelty rend and distort the energy field, thereby creating further distress and discomfort. When you hold gentleness in your energy field, other people, animals, and nature sense this and react warmly. Animals, in particular, sense gentleness within people and respond enthusiastically.

Harmlessness literally involves respecting all living forms and not intentionally harming them in any way. All creatures are part of the divine plan and therefore have a rightful place in creation. Harmlessness means honoring the right of other people, plants, animals, insects, and the earth to coexist in a state of harmony. Sometimes you can be really tested in this regard. Last winter I stayed in an apartment for several days in which rodents also sought reprieve from the harsh winter conditions. Every night they made a ruckus in a storage closet as well as foraged for food in the kitchen. In addition to securing my food supplies, I telepathically requested that they respect my sleeping space. Several months later, upon my return to that apartment, the rodents had departed, probably having returned to their preferred outdoor habitat. I had practiced harmlessness and from that received a surprising feeling of inner gratification.

The power of thought and its impact have already been covered in considerable detail in earlier chapters. Purity of thought, however, relates to the extent to which you are able to perceive the goodness in others. Thinking only positive, accepting, compassionate, and loving thoughts is, without doubt, another challenge. Yet seeing only the beauty and wonder in everything and everyone can be achieved. This is possible when you come to a state of complete self-acceptance and self-love. When you are tolerant, compassionate, and loving toward yourself, you are able to extend the same virtues towards all others. When you are able to say, "Isn't it, he, or she beautiful?" it is because you see in others what you have within. Wishing the very best for others, feeling joy for their achievements, and supporting them unconditionally are other situations where purity of thought is evident. In this state there is no room for jealousy, judgment, or resentment.

It has been my intention to share, however briefly, some of the principles involved in attaining greater spiritual awareness and growth. There are several factors to be mindful of when embarking upon this process.

- When implementing these principles, accept that your intention to change behaviors, attitudes, and thoughts is paramount to achieving success.

- Do not be deterred or feel defeated if at first there appears to be little or no evidence of results. My experience has been that it takes time to have conscious awareness of change.

- Any change experienced is generally subtle and, even if it manifests immediately, is not evident on the conscious and physical levels for possibly months later.

- Often changes are only obvious upon reflection. This becomes evident when previous conditions and situations seem to have disappeared or have changed in a positive manner.

- Persistence and perseverance are essential to producing outcomes that are beneficial for well-being.

- In time the practice of these principles becomes ingrained and normal, and with that further refinement and improvement occurs naturally, as spirit guidance is always readily available to extend your inner growth.

Disconnecting Energetically

On an energy level you connect with people, places, and issues throughout your life journey as they impact on you, whether in a positive or negative manner. Through this means of connection, you literally have an invisible band or cord of energy attached to them. Personal relationships and friendships invoke strong energy cords, and these accumulate over a lifetime. Relationships and friendships do not always continue, yet even after they have ended there remains the energy of that connection and with that the attachment continues.

Have you ever wondered why feelings of guilt, shame, anger, indecision, and so on continue to exist long after a situation, relationship, or friendship has ended? The forgiveness process is, without doubt, instrumental in achieving healing as it promotes feelings of inner peace and completion. Another important process is to release the energy cords of connection. There are several reasons for this.

- Energy cords clutter up the energy field. The memory of attachments from all lifetimes remains within your energy field for as long as you choose to hold onto them.

- Undertaking the process of releasing energy cords regularly assists in keeping the energy field clear and results in feelings of lightness and clarity.

- Releasing the energy cords of attachment results in the release of old emotions of guilt, shame, anger, indecision, and so on.

When attached to another person via energy cords, there is a commingling of emotions.

- You have free will regarding whom you choose to be attached to. As you move through your life journey, you choose friends and relationships that are meaningful and satisfying. The same principle can be applied to energy connections.

- Being attached energetically through many lifetimes can drain your vitality. Detaching the cords can literally revitalize your energy field and result in increased energy levels for daily needs.

The steps involved in disconnecting energetically are straightforward. There are several aspects to be aware of when doing this. Always honor the other person in communication. Be gentle and considerate. Treat the process as a ceremony and hold the intention of honor and sacredness. I prefer the method below, as it is simple, it works, and can easily be applied to any situation.

- Call in the energy of the person. Do this by asking for them by name. You may need to do this more than once. However, you will get a sense of their presence as you will feel their energy vibration or signature.

- Communicate with them as if they were present. Thank them for being part of your life; thank them for whatever is relevant. Then communicate that it is time for a separation of ways and indicate you will be cutting the cords of attachment.

- The next step involves visualizing. If you are unable to visualize, imagine you can "see" the process as you proceed. The results will be the same as it is the intention that creates the scenario.

- Begin by visualizing the cord that is attached to you and extends to the other person. Gently cut it with scissors and then imbed a particle of gold energy into either end of the cord to seal it. When this is done, retract your end of the cord and integrate it into your energy field.

- Finally, thank that person and bless them.

Friends and clients have shared stories where energy cords of attachment have been severed without gentleness, resulting in distressed emotions and reactions of the person on the receiving end. One story clearly demonstrates the importance of consideration and gentleness. A woman disconnected energetically from a former boyfriend. As she did this, she clearly heard, "Ow! Why did you do that?" At that time he lived several states away, though it sounded as though he was standing beside her. Even when the cords are cut with gentleness, the process registers with the recipient on some level.

Given that there is a multitude of connections experienced in all lifetimes, it can become an onerous task to undergo this process and to clear each energy connection one by one. The process can be simplified by finding a quiet space, preferably after completing a meditation, and literally having a mass clearing. Be specific about your intention. Ask your spirit guides to cut all cords of attachment from all times, all planes, and all dimensions that are no longer for your highest good and that do not come from a place of unconditional love. The process only takes a few seconds so remain in the quiet space while it is occurring. When this is done, you will feel lighter and clearer. It must be mentioned that you continue to form energy connections throughout daily interactions, so the process of disconnection needs to be undertaken from time to time.

Protecting Your Space

Just as you connect energetically with people through emotions, relationships, and attachments, you also attract energies that are not necessarily in alignment with your highest good. Many clients share stories of their sensitivity to other people's energies. They know that certain people drain their energy. They also often feel extremely uncomfortable in certain places or with specific people. In such situations it is most likely there is a mismatch of energies, where the energy of the individual does not resonate with the surrounding energies. At times it may even feel as if an attack is occurring energetically. Such situations cause distress to the individual and can leave them feeling powerless and emotionally stressed.

The more you work with positive intent and loving compassion and release negativity from your energy field, the brighter and warmer the energy field vibrates. It becomes healthy and vital and therefore is like a magnet that attracts other energies wishing to share this light energy. I regularly teach clients a simple routine for protecting their energy field. After all, when people have worked diligently to release stored negativity and blockages, they deserve to maintain a clear energy field, free of contamination from other energy sources.

Some years ago I questioned the need to protect the energy field, as this surely would indicate inner fear. My spiritual guidance had consistently urged me to undertake daily protection practice, and in response to my questioning they shared this pearl of wisdom. They pointed out that I would never contemplate leaving the doors and windows in my house open to all that may decide to enter. This is true as I choose whom I invite into my space. They then pointed out that choosing to not practice protection of my being was literally extending an open invitation to all energies to enter my energy field. I got their point, and, since then, have no reservation in sharing the various protection strategies my spiritual guidance have demonstrated.

There are many forms of protection, each equally valid and applicable. As a beginning strategy I suggest that you visualize a bubble of bright light surrounding your whole body (including your energy field) daily and that this bubble acts as a barrier to all negative energy. Visualizing a white bubble takes a fraction of a second. Silently give thanks for the protection it extends.

As your energy field becomes clearer (it has more light), you will attract stronger energies and a simple bubble protection may not suffice. During my journey I have been guided to many different protections and will share some of those.

- Place yourself, your house and property, your car, and animals within a bubble of light.
- When you are in a place that feels discordant to your energies, visualize a bubble of light being placed around other people and

places. Silently affirm that you send them love. Remember, you are coming from a place of love, not of fear!

- Begin by visualizing a bubble of white light around yourself. Then place the bubble within a larger golden pyramid. While doing this, communicate with your spirit guides that you are seeking stronger protection and, if even more is needed, ask that it be given. Also ask that you be shown how to do this. You will be amazed at how readily your spirit guides accede to your request.

- If you readily feel the emotion of other people and are extremely sensitive to energies, you may wish to put in place another form of protection. This one will shield you while it does not limit your ability to continually be a transmitter of unconditional love. Ask that a filter be placed around your energy field. Specify that this filter will allow you to emit the energy of compassion and love while blocking other people's emotions and negative energies.

- When you sense the barbs of thoughts and emotions from other people, ask that these be returned to the sender with love. Whatever is sent to you, whether with love or malice, can always be returned with the energy of love.

Having a clear energy field creates more energy and enhances well-being. When the energy field is bright and unaffected by the influence of other energies, this supports the process of achieving a state of non-attachment. As you undertake the process of cutting the energy cords of attachment and ensure your energy field is clean, you will feel less emotional and uncertain. If anything, you achieve greater clarity regarding how you can be of service to others while simultaneously honoring what your soul is seeking.

CHAPTER TWENTY-FIVE
Know
Yourself

*"We can easily forgive a child
who is afraid of the dark;
the real tragedy of life is
when men are afraid of the light."*
—Plato—

A factor involved in achieving good health and well-being lies in striving to reconnect with the essence of your soul. When you tune into the frequency of your soul, you radiate its life force. This is the light referred to in previous chapters. It is the luminescence of your energy field from which you have cleared stored emotions and blockages from not only this lifetime but from many others.

In this chapter I will focus on the differences between the external perception of self and the real or inner self that is submerged and hidden from view. By reading this book and undertaking the suggested strategies and exercises, you should by now have an awareness that you are not merely the exterior that is presented to the world. The real inner you is pure energy. This energy has intelligent consciousness that is far superior to the ego consciousness that is used as a vehicle for operating in a physical reality. Reconnecting with the essence of who you are is critical to creating and maintaining wellness and balance in your life. The inner self, or soul, is contained within the energy field. It is this that seeks to release the limitations and blockages that have prevented you from seeing the inner beauty you hold.

Undertaking spiritual and religious practice, including prayer and meditation, is not sufficient on its own to ensure balance and wellness. A quick assessment of the continuing conflicts in world affairs is an indication that globally we are still far from truly being healed, irrespective of the millions of people worldwide who undertake religious practice and meditate daily.

On a superficial level most people are able to define who and what they are by their status within society, by employment classification, and by public persona. It is common to portray an image of yourself as being highly successful, financially stable, a competent parent, or whatever else you choose to create. It is easy to base your status within a societal framework on assessment and judgment. For example, it is common practice to identify your strengths and weaknesses in an employment context. That identification is then carried through to a belief system you hold about yourself and a wider reality. It is easy to believe you are what you portray! Though it is preferable to portray positive aspects, especially those that are socially accepted and valued, inherent insecurities will surface usually when they are least expected. Insecurities and perceived weaknesses are often due to the fact that there has not been full exploration and healing of an aspect of your character. Nevertheless, once you define and internalize a certain belief, you demonstrate its truth in many ways.

Socrates is supposedly reported to have responded, "Know yourself" when asked how the meaning of life can be found. What does "know yourself" mean? This does not mean being able to clearly articulate faults, virtues, likes, dislikes, strengths, and weaknesses. Using a debit and credit rating scale to assess your life involves subjective assessment and judgment and is not the most reliable determinant of your inner essence. Your personal characteristics are the outer coating or layer; they are the ones you have chosen and created for experiencing life. This outer coating is somewhat like donning a suit. The suit may look smart, fit well, and enhance other physical attributes. What it does not do, however, is reveal what is really underneath. It does not reveal what is at the very core of the person wearing it. The suit only disguises what is on an inner or deeper level.

Knowing yourself means coming to know the truth and essence of who you are. This is the soul that resides within everyone. It is this essence that becomes submerged under the many suits or masks that are worn in daily interactions. Your soul is an integral part of everything that is experienced in life. It has consciousness that exerts itself through various means. It is normal to become oblivious to its presence and real impact upon your life, due to the demands of an entrenched, dominant reality.

The soul clamors to be felt and heard in everything you do. It will also show its resistance to what you are doing in many ways. This can be through experiencing feelings of guilt, by manifesting as some form of illness, or through emotional and mental turbulence. Whenever there is any sign of discomfort or pain in life, it's a signal that the soul is expressing its distress. It is a sign that life is not lived in alignment with what is for your highest good.

A large component of living meaningfully and in undertaking a spiritual journey is to reconnect with your soul and to integrate it fully into every aspect of your physical reality. The outer layers—perceptions, beliefs, ego consciousness—happily obscure your soul and allow it little voice. Competing demands for your attention happily divert you from giving thought and time to finding your way back to the core of your essence. Not only that, these competing demands cleverly shroud the way; they create barriers and distractions to block you from discovering this truth!

Going within literally involves becoming reacquainted with your soul. You were fully acquainted and connected when you incarnated, but the mere fact of living a physical life means that you become encapsulated within the dominant paradigms. Our scientific and rational way of living and viewing the world focuses on the externals and on what is verifiable and rational. This is not how it has always been. Traditional cultures and societies understood and honored the soul and its integral place in the whole cosmic universe. As society moves away from the time-honored traditional beliefs and accepts the currently held scientific paradigms as the only truth, the alienation from soul intensifies. Luckily, however, your soul has intent and a voice. It lets you know in many ways when there is an aspect of yourself that is not being honored. It reminds you that life is meant to be lived in alignment with your inner purpose.

A wise man once offered sound advice that opened my eyes to the subtle messages my soul was attempting to convey. All of my endeavors to create a career in the corporate world were continually met with resistance. This was in spite of all the goal setting and strategic planning I had implemented. It seemed as though doors of opportunity would close whenever I eagerly attempted to walk through them. This wise man stated that whenever attempts continually meet resistance, you are being diverted toward the correct direction. Nowadays I give gratitude for those closed doors. My soul has plans for me that are still unfolding!

Your soul always knows what is in your best interests, even when you can't see or sense it. Sometimes drastic measures are taken in order that the message is received. A friend was always rushing through life; it seemed as if there was never enough time. It was not surprising to learn that he had been involved in a minor car accident. This accident seemed to be a clear message for him to slow down, but he didn't heed it. Not long afterward an incident resulted in foot damage, which forced him to slow down.

Messages or signs come in many ways. You can choose to heed them, make changes in your life that are in alignment with the purpose of your soul, or you can ignore them. The soul does not give up—it continues sending out signs regardless of any conscious life choices. Ultimately, ignoring the signs results in pain or distress to some extent. There is another aspect to this element of life consequences that has not been discussed and that is the universal law of karma, otherwise known as cause and effect. Even when a condition of ill health is karmically induced, practicing positive intent and working with the attributes of selflessness, love, and service provides an opportunity to reduce the karmic debt and will result in healing on many levels.

You may wonder why it is important to reconnect with your soul. Your soul is the essence of who you really are and is vastly different to the outer layers of existence you create. Reconnecting with your soul involves learning to recognize the many signs and messages that are continually delivered. These come in many forms, and I will describe some, as they may be helpful:

- Listen to the inner voice of intuition. This comes in different ways for people. Only you will come to know the means by which your inner spirit communicates its messages. You literally don't have to do anything except listen in order to know how to best respond. It sounds easy but given that the world is usually filled with noisy distractions it is normal to miss the soft whisperings or subtle signs that come at unexpected times.

- Respond to the voice of intuition. When you are given a message, heed it and respond accordingly. The voice of intuition is your inner guidance. It expresses what is really needed.

- When confronted with a choice in any situation, respond according to how you initially feel inwardly. It will feel like there is a soft and quiet nudging to take a specific option or direction. This is gut instinct or intuition.

- Logic usually presents a rational choice after the gut instinct makes it presence felt, and this is a sign that the mind has stepped in to offer a practical response. The logical choice is based on what has worked and been safe in past situations and does not necessarily reflect the best choice in any current situation. How often do you hear people say, "If only I had listened to my initial instinct"? This is a common reaction when following the practical mind responses. The mind delights in providing safe responses and overrides any inner creative urges.

• Learn to trust your instinct. Respond to its strong messages, and in time it will become second nature to live life in this manner.

• Listening to the inner voice will bring about changes and opportunities that would not otherwise occur. It opens the door to knowing and accepting who you are and what you really want to be and do, and not necessarily what you think is the case.

• Observe coincidences. Nothing in the universe ever occurs randomly. There is a reason for everything. Coincidences are another means by which your soul provides information. It becomes a matter of recognizing the synchronicity and opportune moments as they arise and then responding accordingly.

• Allow time for quiet and reflection. Be aware of the thoughts that surface unbidden as they provide further information from your soul. The moments when this is likely to occur are just prior to sleep and upon first awakening before mind consciousness surfaces.

Sometimes the messages are missed but the soul is forgiving and determined. It will persist, and so they will come in other ways. Being aware and mindful of signs and messages is a wonderful way of becoming acquainted with the real you. The more this is practiced, the easier it becomes to see the meanings and connections, and there is greater scope for making choices that enrich life opportunities. Sometimes, in life, events just flow beautifully with little individual effort or concentration. This is known as being in the flow; it also indicates clear alignment between soul purpose and physical direction.

Being mindful of what feels right and acting accordingly will strengthen the connection with your soul. However, certain life situations present dilemmas and inner stress. One of these is the influence of peer pressure. Often the desire to be accepted overrides deep inner knowing about what feels right and appropriate. When you feel pressured into saying and behaving in ways that do not feel comfortable, your soul is not honored. Feelings of guilt and regret indicate behaviors and emotions that are not aligned with soul purpose. When that little inner voice says "no" to actions involving peer pressure or to any other behavior, learn to heed that "no" and honor it. You will immediately feel lighter and happier. Having said "no" the first time makes it easier to use that hugely powerful word in the future. This action is also about speaking and living your truth. It means that your soul truth is reflected in what you say, do, and think on the physical level.

Sometimes speaking your truth will cause difficulty in communication and personal interactions, especially when first attempting this. Family, friends and colleagues may have discomfort in hearing this change in tone and intent. Instead of complying with their wishes, you are taking responsibility for your needs and honoring what feels right. At all times be gentle with others, even when responding firmly. In honoring what feels appropriate, your words and actions can be perceived as being threatening. This is because others see and feel a change within you, and this creates inner distress for them. Suddenly their perception of reality is challenged, especially when things do not go as planned. However, the more you live according to your soul truth, the easier life becomes. In many ways, obstacles no longer become prominent, and moments of peace become commonplace. When your soul is happy, it will be reflected in your physical life.

Let go of preconceived ideas about how life is meant to be lived and instead allow life to be as it is. Accept what is happening right now as being perfect. Even if you have debt, health problems, or employment difficulties, there are still many beautiful things happening every day. Acknowledge and give gratitude for whatever you have, including difficulties, as these challenges are powerful teachers. If you have debt issues, then this is a chance to learn how to manage your finances better in order to become debt free. Health problems offer an opportunity to take responsibility for creating wellness. In every challenge there exists a silver lining. Endeavor to find that silver lining. Your soul understands exactly what is happening and the reasons for the difficulty. Instead, view challenge as a time of great learning. Your soul is here to learn and grow. All difficulties present this prospect!

Adversity is an opportunity for growth and empowerment in your experience of life. When working consciously with your soul's purpose you have the opportunity for increased awareness and mastery in all aspects of life. This ultimately results in meaningful inner and outer changes, as the two seem to mesh into one in new and exciting ways. This literally means that the external and inner realities integrate and harmonize as a shared reality. There is no longer any separation or duality. The outer reflects the inner and the inner, likewise, is reflected outward in all situations.

Know that you are co-creator of your life and possess the power to create life in ways previously unimagined. The power to do so lies within. Your soul will happily assist in creating affirmative changes based on intent and aligned with your real self, and not on an external image. As you strive to find deeper meaning to life, it is inevitable that reconnection with your soul occurs gradually. However, any penchant you have for criticism and negativity must be overcome in order to feel the love that emanates from your soul. When the reconnection occurs, you literally find the energy of unconditional love within. Not surprisingly, once it is found you also come to recognize it within everyone and everything else. Coming to feel, know, and accept this as another aspect of the journey within. And once this has been integrated fully into the energy field, the spiritual and physical reality blend joyously and harmoniously into a unified oneness.

Coming to know yourself is a journey back to the essence of self or soul. This is what going within means. It literally means coming to understand that the inner knowing is what gives you purpose and is really who you are in essence. The soul is stunningly beautiful. It does not judge or see imperfections. Your soul is your connection with the Creator. It is also the essence of the Divine Spirit within you. When you live according to the dictates of your soul, this radiates outward from your physical being. The nourished and honored soul lights up the energy field. Living positively, with loving intent and in service to humanity, strengthens the energy field and provides additional fuel to the soul. It is a congruent intermingling and coexistence of energies. It is this harmonious balance of energies that ultimately generates healing and wellness.

Luminescent Reflection (Refer to CD)

Have you ever really looked at yourself and seen the inherent beauty you possess? This visualization exercise fosters an appreciation and feeling of inner beauty. Practice this several times until you feel comfortable with the process, and you may then choose to modify it so that it is personalized. You know your unique qualities. This exercise offers you the opportunity to fully acknowledge your uniqueness.

Sit comfortably in a chair with your back straight, your legs uncrossed, and your feet on the floor. Rest your arms gently on your lap. Close your eyes and breathe in deeply and slowly. Exhale gently. Repeat this breath cycle a few times.

Focus all of your attention on your breath. If your breathing is hurried or shallow, change it to be slow and deep. On your inhalation, visualize every part of your body filled with white light. As you exhale, feel your body release stored tension and emotions. Continue breathing deeply and slowly until your muscles are relaxed and your mind is calm.

In this relaxed state, take your consciousness outside your physical body. Visualize a large mirror placed about two feet directly in front of you. The mirror is clear, bright, and trimmed with beautiful gold leaves and vines. Slowly realize the magical properties of this mirror. Everything placed in front of the mirror is revealed. There are no secrets.

Keeping your eyes closed, look at the image in the mirror. What you see is not your physical body. It is your inner essence or your soul. Look closely at your soul reflected in the mirror in front of you. What do you see? Can you see the luminescence of your essence? Is your reflection an orb of golden light? Does your essence have color?

As you observe your inner essence, feel its magnificence. Enjoy its beauty and radiance. If you wish to communicate with your soul, go ahead and freely express your thoughts and feelings. You may hear a response in the form of whispered words inside your head. Accept whatever happens, as you are perfectly safe in the presence of your real self.

Your inner essence is an integral part of who you are. Its inherent beauty remains undimmed, no matter what may happen in your physical reality. You hold this vibrant luminescent energy within you at all times.

When you are ready, return your awareness to your seated body. Feel your revitalizing breath still circulating within your body. Now, with your eyes still closed, look back in the mirror. This time, your physical body is in the reflection, but it is not the physical body that you have seen reflected countless times. Now that you have experienced your inner essence, you will never again see yourself in the same manner. You understand that your physical body provides a home for your inner essence, but this home does not dim what lies within. Your essence radiates within this home. The glow of your inner essence will forever extend beyond your physical body. Feel this glow. Feel its warmth and strength. Observe your physical body with this emanating glow, no longer the physical body you were accustomed to. This reflection is the real you.

Slowly bring your attention back to your breath as you get ready to return to your physical reality. You have uncovered the perfect essence of your being. Feel it radiate into and through your physical body at all times. Hold this image of the nature of your true self in your mind and in your heart. Your inner beauty is always within you. Allow your light to shine in everything you do.

BIBLIOGRAPHY

Brennan, Barbara Ann. *Hands of Light*. Bantam Books, 1998.

Budilovsky, Joan, and Eve Adamson. *The Complete Idiot's Guide to Meditation*. Alpha Books, 2003.

Cabot, Dr. Sandra. *The Liver Cleansing Diet*. Women's Health Advisory Service, 1996.

Cadbury, Deborah. *Altering Eden: The Feminization of Nature*. St. Martin's Press, 1997.

Chomsky, Noam, and Edward S. Herman. *Manufacturing Consent*. Pantheon Press, 1998.

Chopra, Deepak. *How to Know God*. Rider Books, 2000.

Cohen, Alissa. *Living on Live Food*. Cohen Publishing Company, 2004.

Dalai Lama. *Ancient Wisdom, Modern World*. Little, Brown and Company, 1999.

Dalai Lama, and Howard C. Cutler, M.D. *The Art of Happiness*. Riverhead Books, 1988.

Day, Phillip. *Health Wars*. Credence Publications, 2001.

Dean, Carolyn, M.D. N.D., Martin Feldman, M.D., Gary Null, Ph.D., and Debora Rasio, M.D. "Death By Medicine." *Nexus New Times* 11, no. 5.

Derber, Charles. *Corporation Nation: How Corporations Are Taking Over Our Lives—And What We Can Do About It*. St. Martin's Press, 2000.

Dyer, Wayne. *The Power of Intention*. Hay House, Inc., 2004.

Hanley, Jesse Lynn, M.D., and Nancy Deville. *Tired of Being Tired*. Berkley Publishing Group, 2001.

Hay, Louise. *You Can Heal Yourself*. Hay House, Inc., 1984.

Howell, Edward. *Enzyme Nutrition*. Avery Publishing, 1995.

Leadbeater, C. W. *The Chakras*. Theosophical Publishing House, 1927.

Mackenzie, Vicki. *Cave in the Snow*. Bloomsbury, 1998.

Miller, R.A., and I. Miller, "The Schumann's Resonance and Human Psychobiology." *Nexus New Times* 10, no. 3.

Myss, Carolyn. *Energetics of Healing*. VHS. Gemini Sun Records. 2001.

Noontil, Annette. *The Body is the Barometer of the Soul*. McPherson's Printing Group, 1998.

Rojek, Mark. "The Essentials of Enzyme Nutrition Therapy." *Nexus New Times* 10, no. 6.

Saraydarian, Torkom. *New Dimensions in Healing*. T.S.G. Publishing Foundation, Inc., 1992.

Seattle Times, "Strong Warning on Anti-Depressants Urged," September 15, 2004.

Sisson, Colin P. *Inner Adventures*. Total Press Ltd., 1997.

ADDITIONAL REFERENCES

The reader may wish to further explore some of the concepts covered in this book. Below are some references that may be useful.

Alexander, Phillip, N.D. *It Could be Allergy and It Can Be Cured.* Ethicare Pty Ltd., 1990.

Baroody, Dr. Theodore A. *Alkalize or Die.* Holographic Health Press, 1991.

Berkson, D. Lindsay. *Hormone Deception.* Contemporary Books, 2000.

Bryson, Christopher. *The Flouride Deception.* Seven Stories Press, 2004.

Carey, Ken. *Return of the Bird Tribes.* Harper, 1988.

Courteney, Hazel. *Divine Intervention.* Cico Books, 2002.

Cousens, Gabriel, M.D. *Depression Free for Life.* Quill, 2001.

Day, Phillip. *Cancer, Why We're Still Dying to Know the Truth.* Credence Publications, 1999.

—. *The Mind Game.* Credence Publications, 2002.

—. *Food For Thought.* Credence Publications, 2001.

Edward, John. *Crossing Over.* Jodere Group, Inc., 2001.

Flickstein, Matthew. *Swallowing the River Ganges—A Practice Guide to the Path of Purification.* Wisdom Publications, 2001.

Hansen, Bente. *Messages From Beyond—Channeled Messages From the Arcturus Community.* Smallprint, 2001.

Hawkins, David R., M.D., Ph.D. *Power vs. Force.* Hay House, 2002.

Hoffman, Enid. *Develop Your Psychic Skills.* Whitford Press, 1981.

Krishnamurti, J. *Total Freedom—The Essential Krishnamurti.* Harper, 1996.

Lawrence, Felicity. *Not On The Label—What Really Goes into the Food on your Plate.* Penquin, 2004.

Levoy, Greg. *Callings—Finding and Following and Authentic Life.* Three Rivers Press, 1997.

Maclaine, Shirley. *The Camino—A Journey of the Spirit.* Pocket Books, 2000.

Medical Research Associates. *The Encyclopedia of Medical Breakthroughs & Forbidden Treatments.* Medical Research Associates LLC, 2005.

O'Donnell, Ken. *Pathways to Higher Consciousness.* Eternity Ink, Brahma Kumaris Raja Yoga, 1996.

Page, Linda. *Healthy Healing.* Traditional Wisdom, Inc., 2003.

Rasha. *Oneness-The Teachings.* Jodere Group, 2003.

Ricketson, Susan Cooley. *The Dilemma of Love.* 2000.

Roads, Michael J. *More Than Money, True Prosperity: A Wholistic Guide To Having It All.* SilverRoads Publishing, 2003.

Roman, Sanaya. *Spiritual Growth, Being Your Higher Self.* HJ Kramer, Inc., 1989.

Roman, Sanaya, and Duane Packer. *Opening to Channel—How To Connect With Your Guide.* HJ Kramer, Inc., 1987.

Saraydarian, H. trans. *The Bhagavad Gita.* Aquarian Educational Group, 1974.

Saraydarian, Torkom. *Thought and the Glory of Thinking.* T.S.G. Publishing Foundation, Inc., 1996.

Tolle, Eckhart. *The Power of Now—A Guide to Spiritual Enlightenment.* Namaste Publishing, 1999.

Trudeau, Kevin. *Natural Cures "They" Don't Want You To Know About.* Alliance Publishing Group, 2004.

Walker, Martin J. *Skewed: Psychiatric Hegemony and the Manufacture of Mental Illness.* Slingshot Publications Ltd., 2003.

Whitaker, Julian, M.D. *Dr. Whitaker's Guide to Natural Healing.* Prima Publishing, 1995.